Illustrated Guide
- to -
Canine Anatomy

First Edition

Published by: Kevin C. Stevens

Design, Layout, and Illustrations by Kevin Stevens

Library and Archives of Canada in Publication

ISBN: 978-1-7382014-1-9

First Edition

KS Design/Publishing

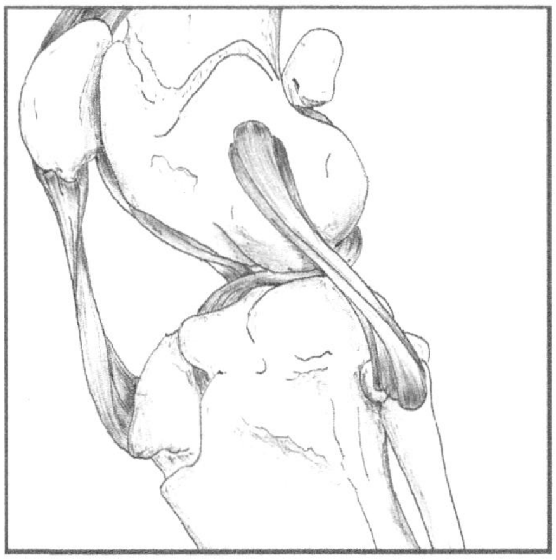
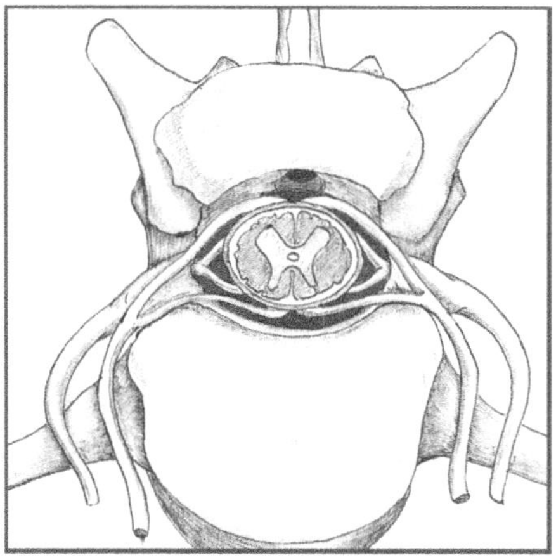
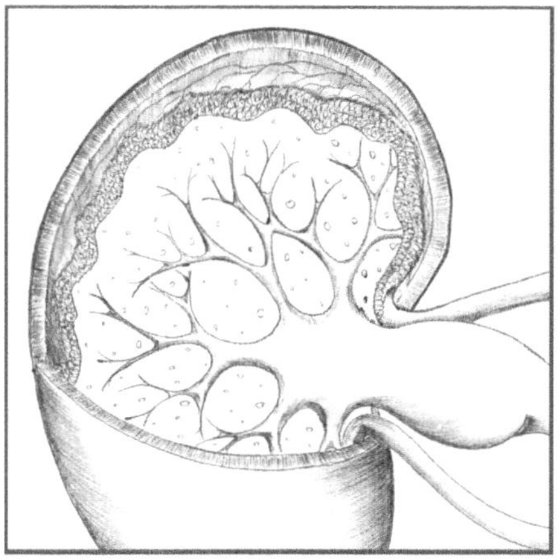
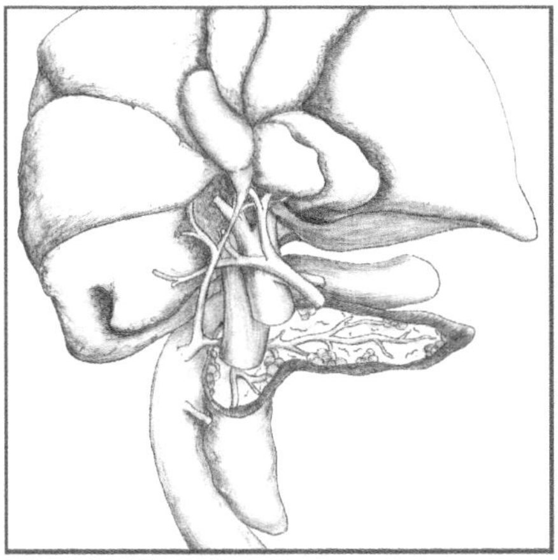
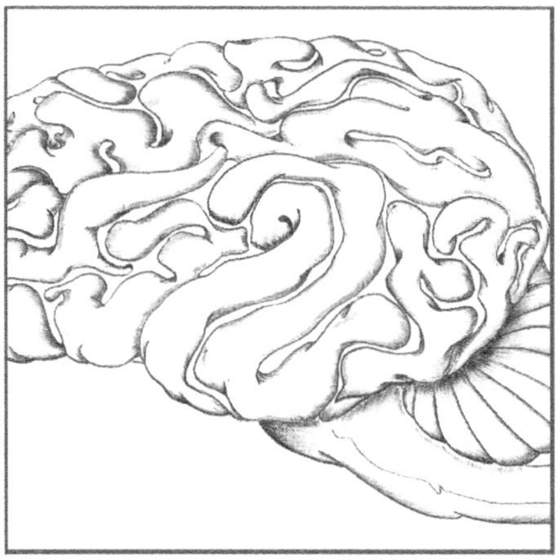
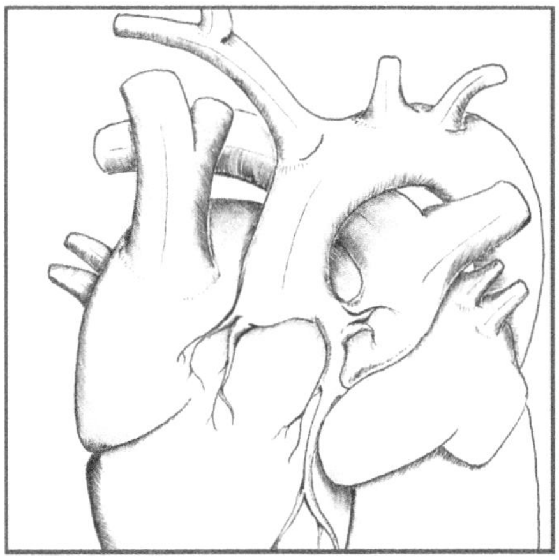
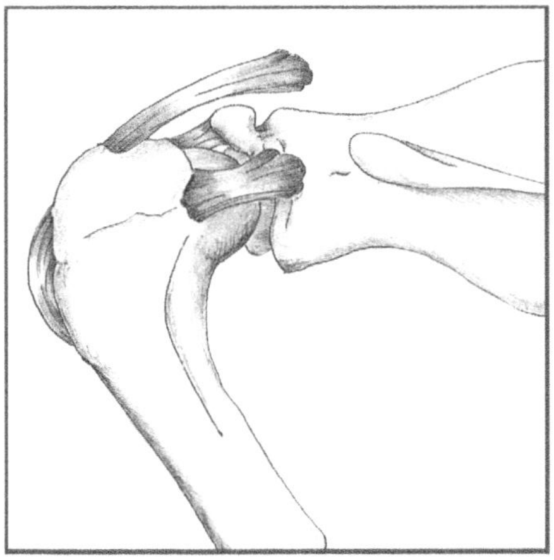
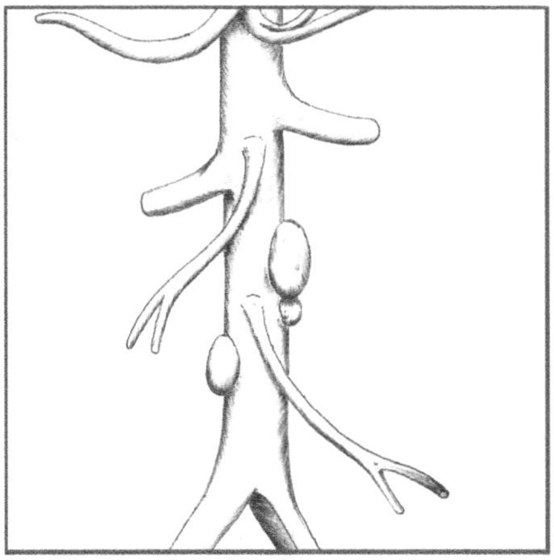
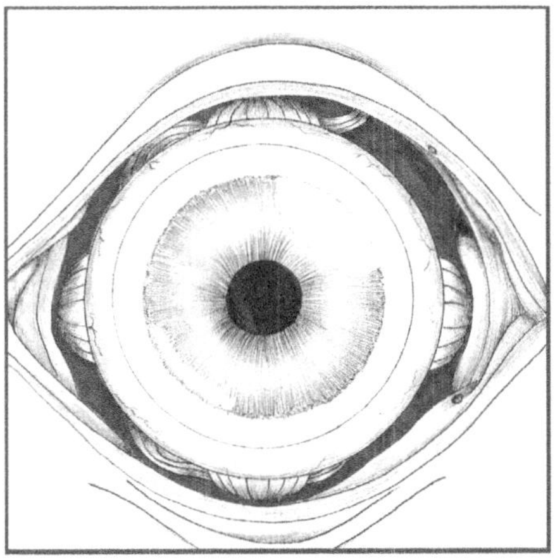

- ILLUSTRATED GUIDE TO -

CANINE ANATOMY

Kevin Stevens

Introduction

Do we need another anatomy book?

Honestly, we don't. There are so many great anatomy books already out there that it can be difficult to decide which ones to include in your library. Over the years I have found that when you need information you need it quickly and don't always have the luxury of searching through an encyclopedia of anatomy.

This project started with a few hand drawn sketches to help explain structural neurological anatomy to a colleague. I got a little carried away with it, and it quickly started growing into something more (though I never expected an actual book).

I hope you enjoy this book and that it finds a home in your library. It may be the anatomy book you never needed but I hope it is one that you can't live without.

- Kevin Stevens

Acknowledgments

Thank you to everyone that made this book possible. My colleagues, friends, and family for recognizing the potential in a few drawings and encouraging me in this project. To those that spent hours reading, proofing, and editing my work, I am truly grateful.

- Kevin

Preface

How to use this book

This is not the first or most comprehensive anatomy book ever made and that is entirely on purpose. I have intentionally simplified the amount of information, keeping it to the anatomy that you're likely to use on a regular basis. I have included places for additional notes and I've even started you off with a few basic pieces of information.

I encourage you to use this book in whatever way suits you the best. Write in it, color the pictures, add extra notes, and use the blank pictures to quiz yourself. Think of it more as an anatomy journal than a text book.

However you choose, I hope this book supports your knowledge of canine anatomy whether you are a seasoned professional or just beginning your career in veterinary medicine.

Contents

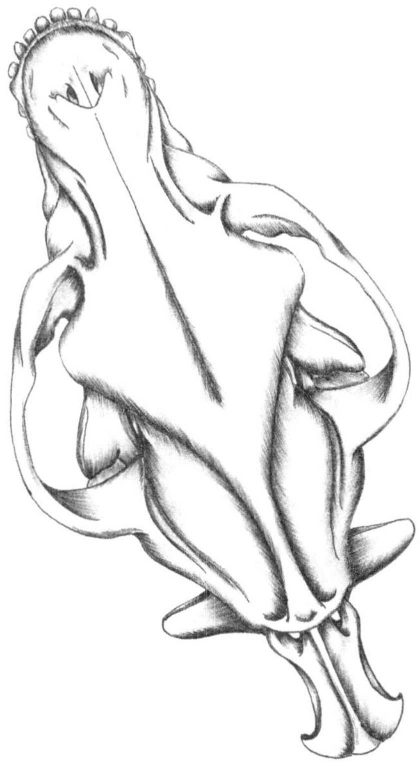

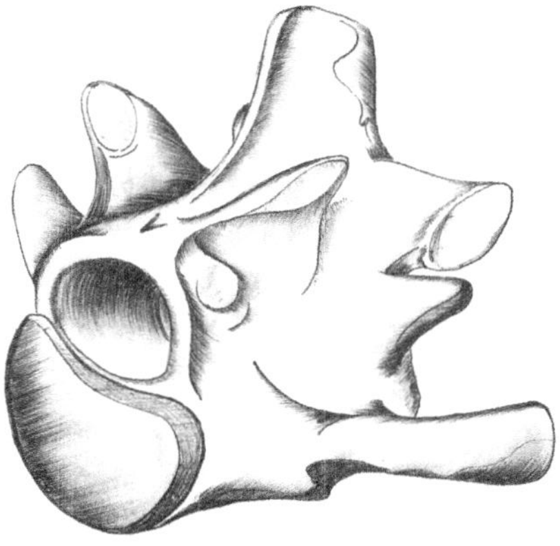

Contents

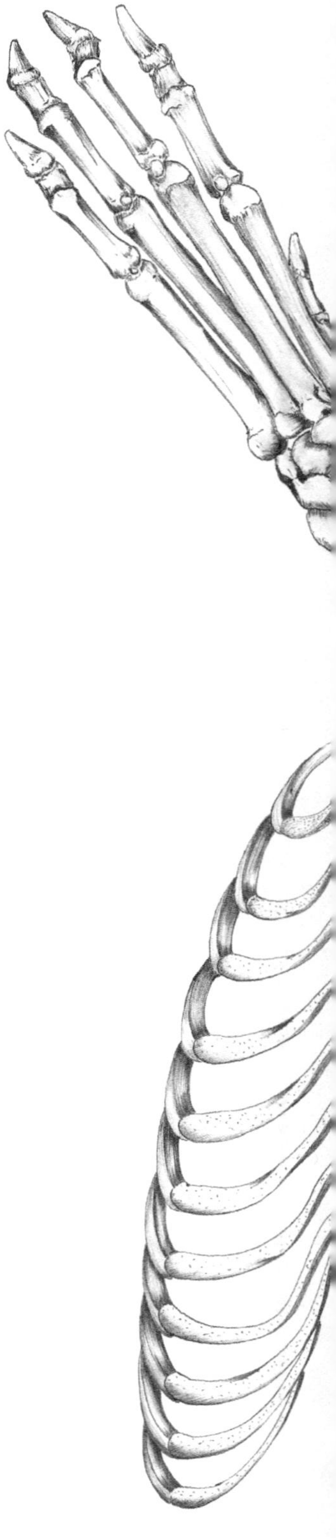

the Head

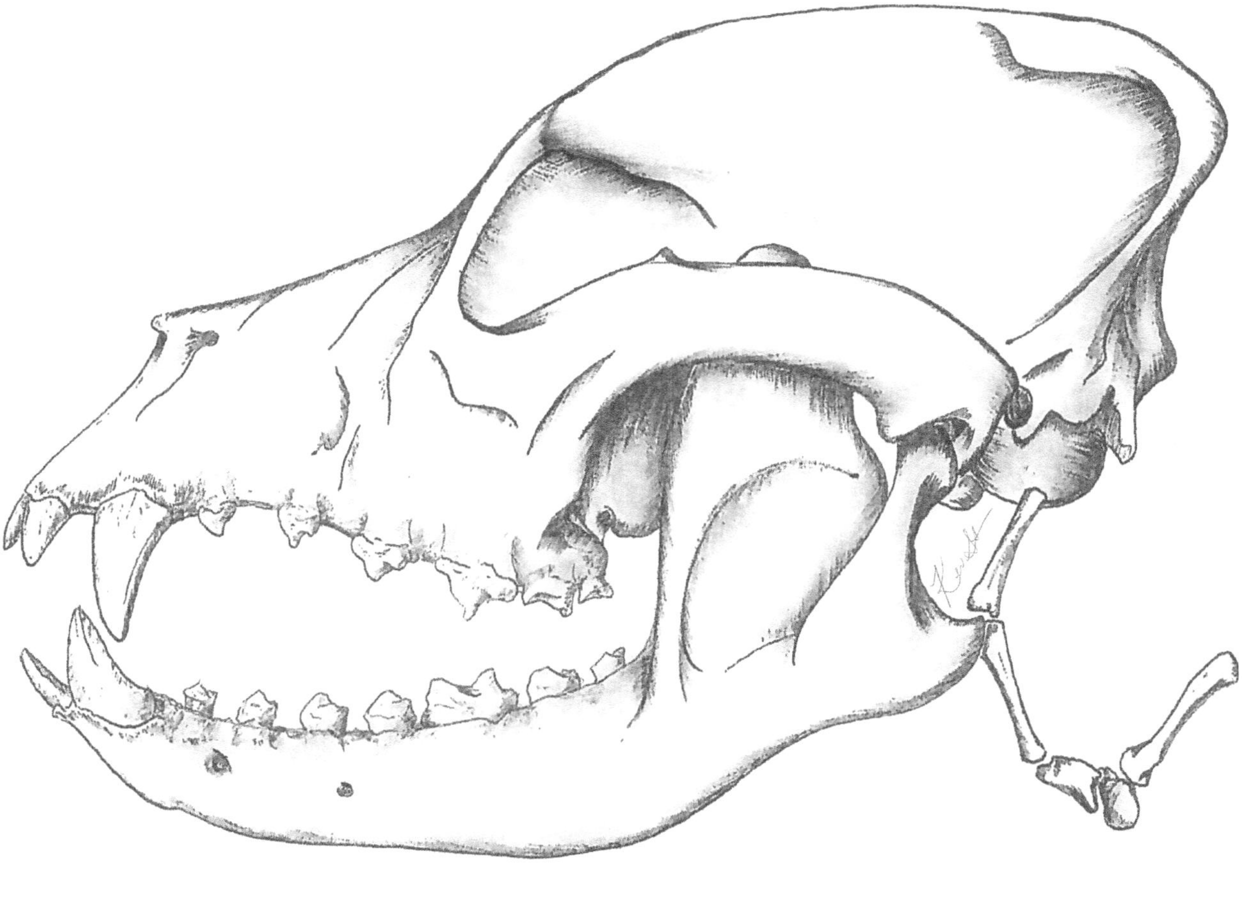

Notes:

- The skull is made up of approximately 50 bones.
- The boney protuberance on the top of a dog's skull is called the occiput or occipital protuberance.
- Dogs have 42 teeth; 20 Maxillary teeth: 6 incisors, 2 canines, 8 premolars and 4 molars. 22 Mandibular teeth: 6 incisors, 2 canines, 8 premolars, and 6 molars.
- There are 4 ventricles in the brain, each containing a choroid plexus which produce cerebrospinal fluid.
- CSF (cerebrospinal fluid) surrounds and protects the brain and spinal cord.
- White matter is responsible for transmitting signals.
- Grey matter is responsible for processing information.
- The head includes 4 sinuses, the Maxillary, Frontal, Ethmoid, and Sphenoid.
- The spinal cord exits the skull through an opening called the foramen magnum.
- There are 12 cranial nerve pairs in the head.

Skull: Lateral View

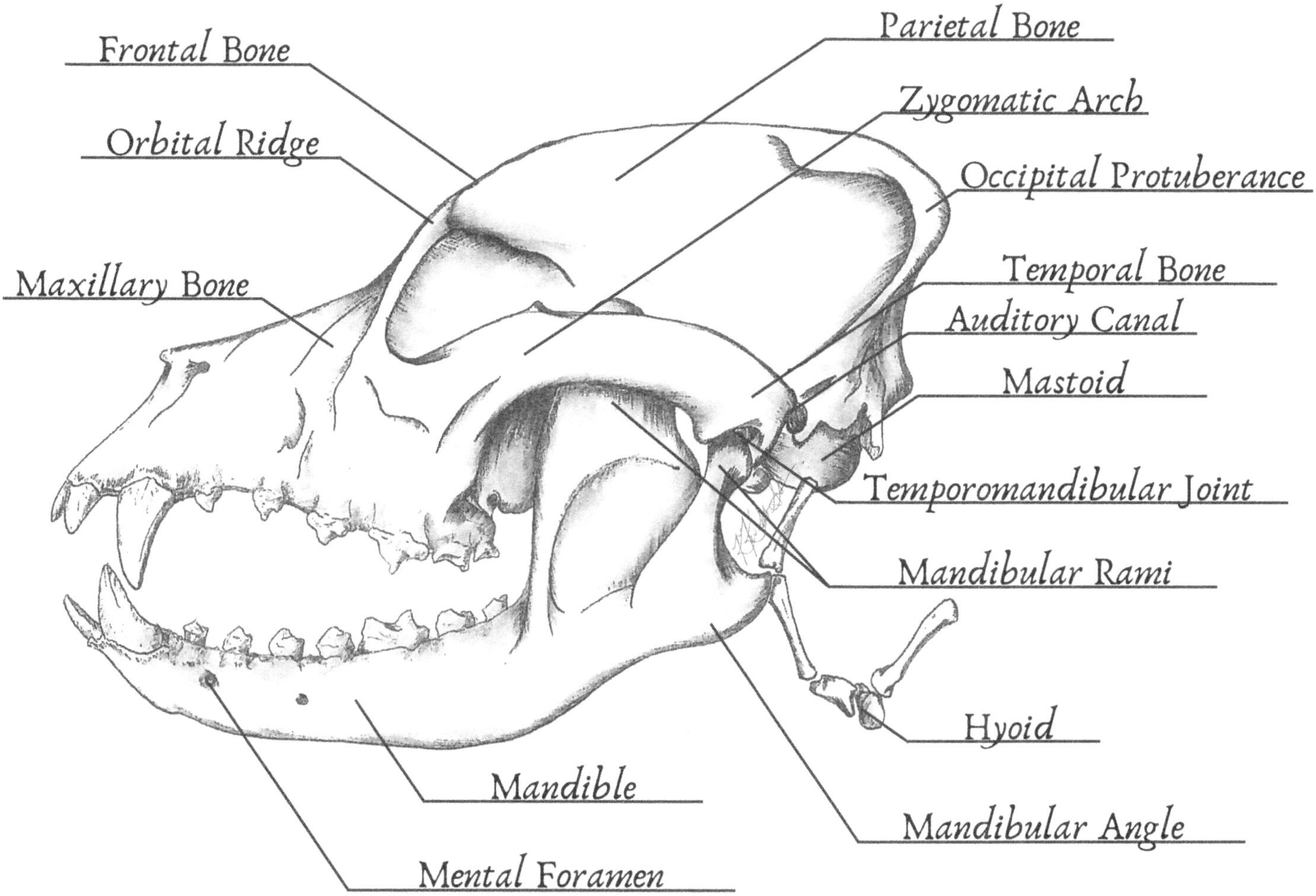

Skull: Lateral View

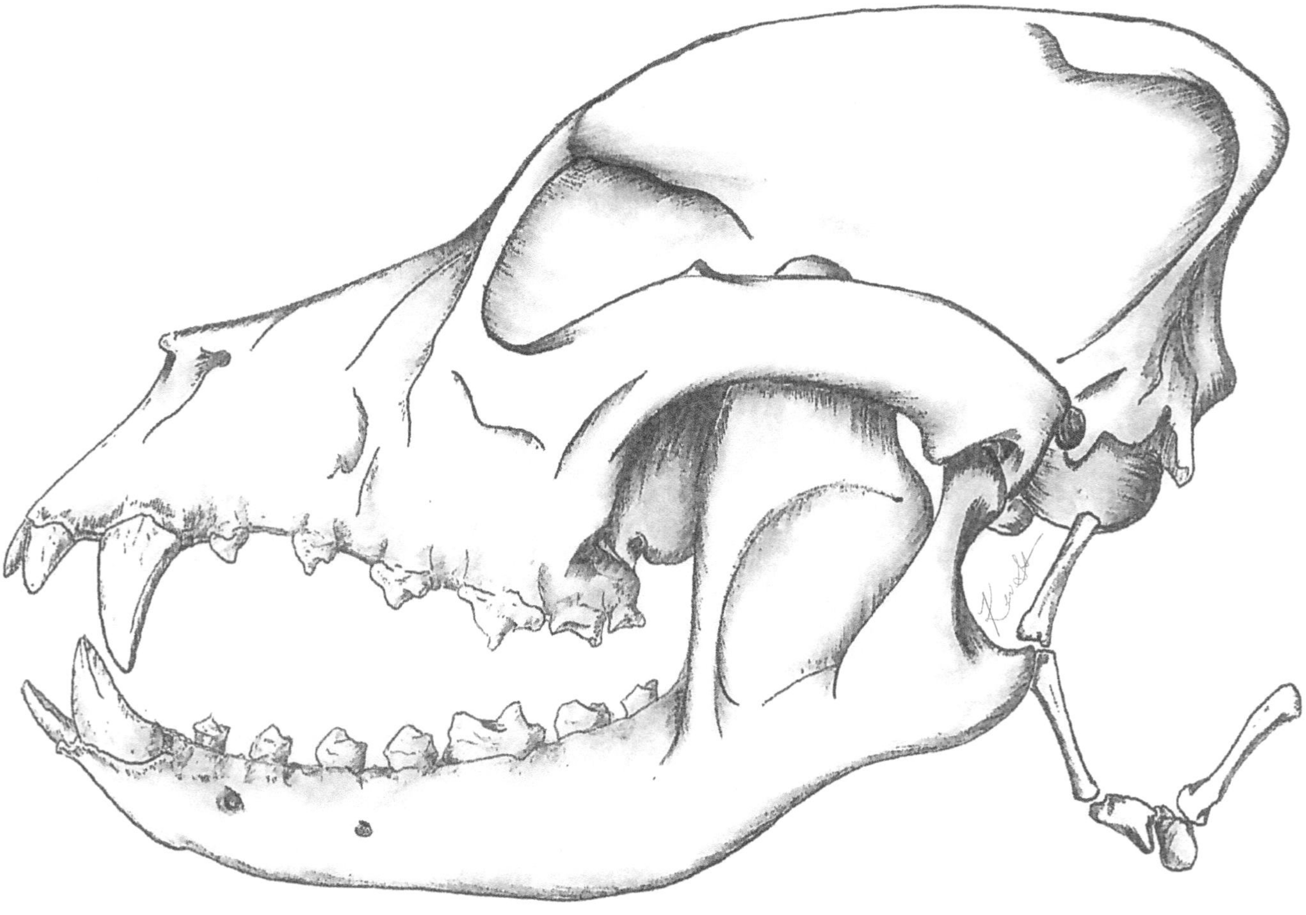

Skull: Superior View

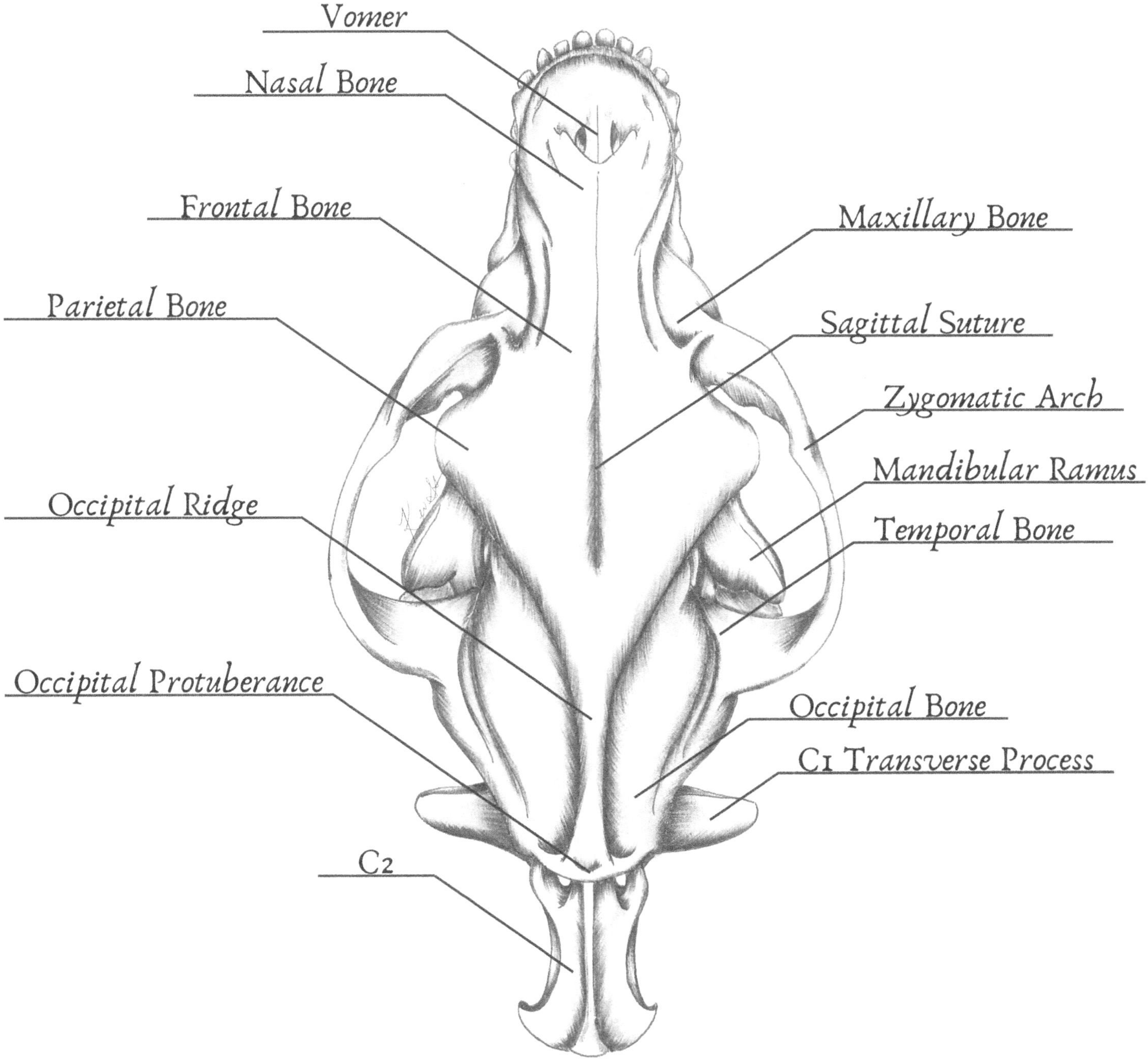

Skull: Superior View

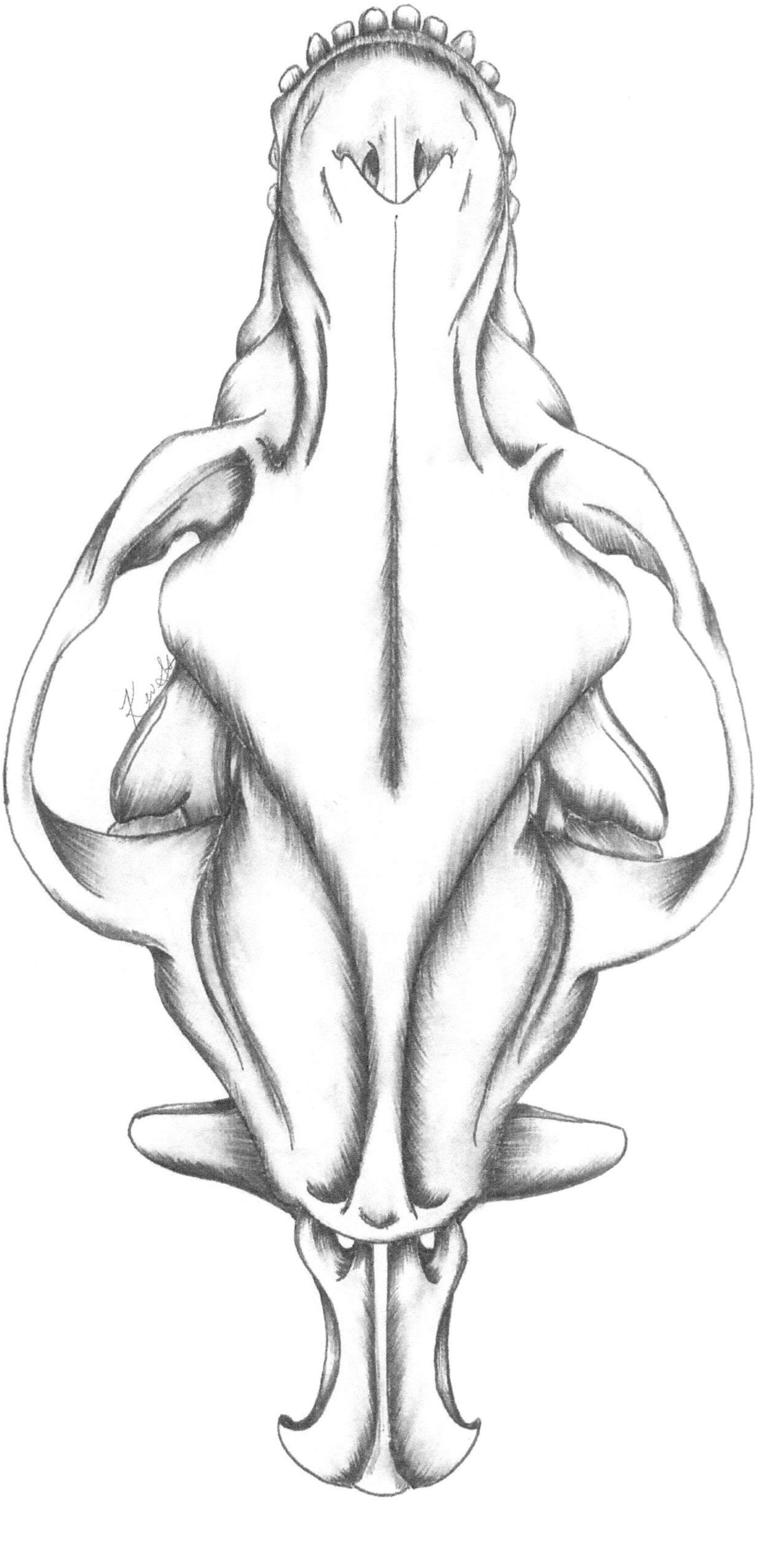

Head: Mid Sagittal

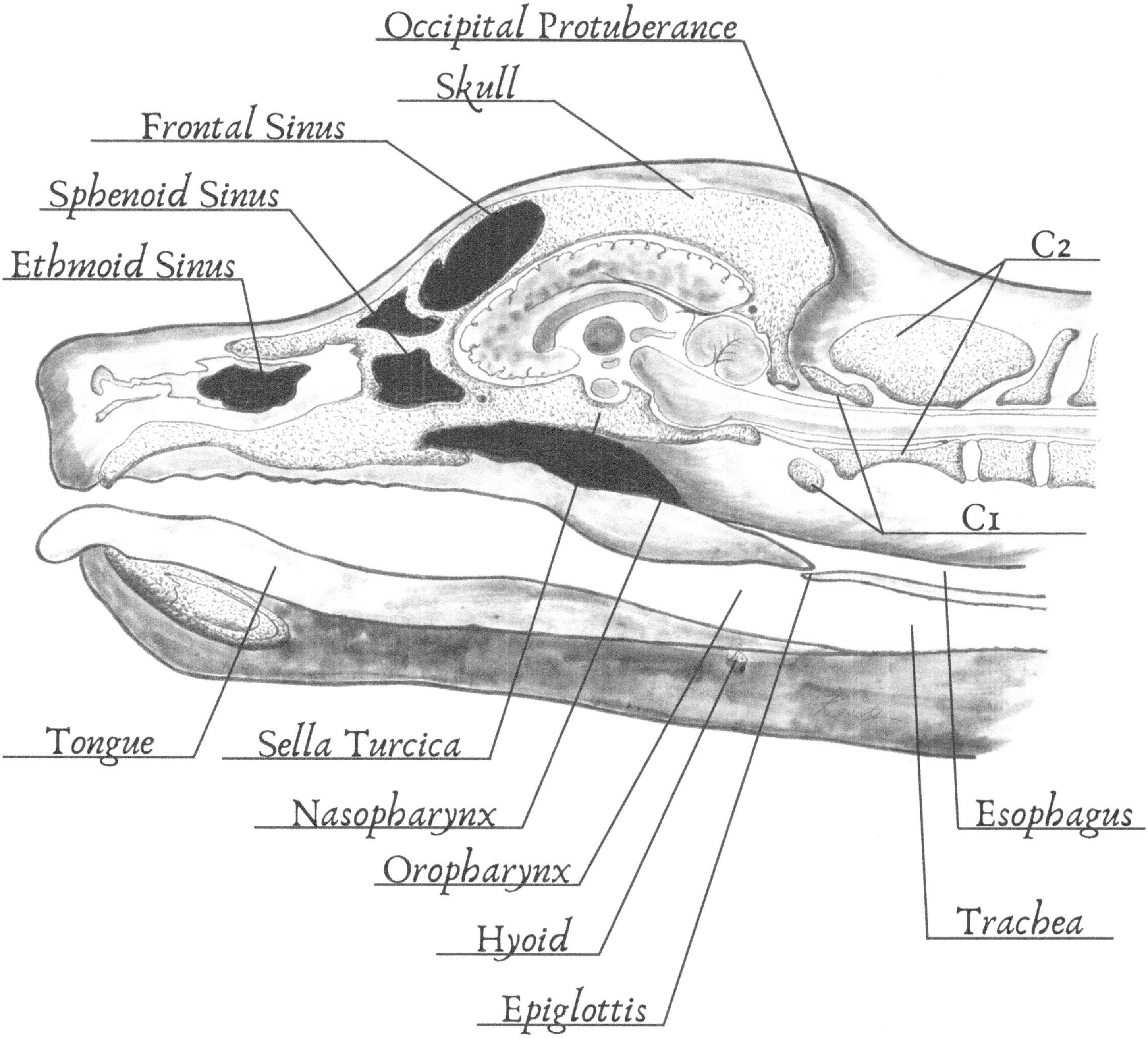

Head: Mid Sagittal

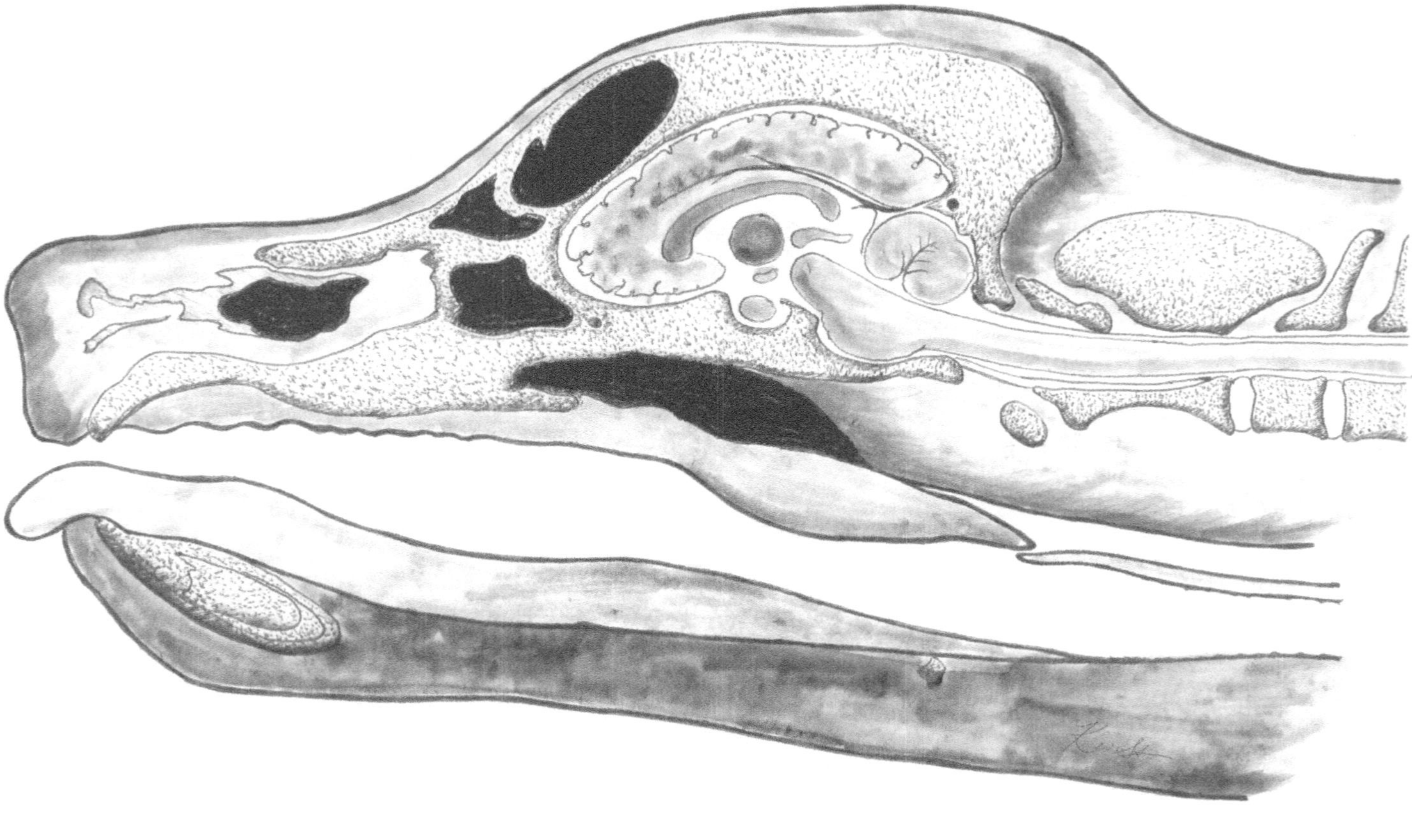

Brain: Lateral View

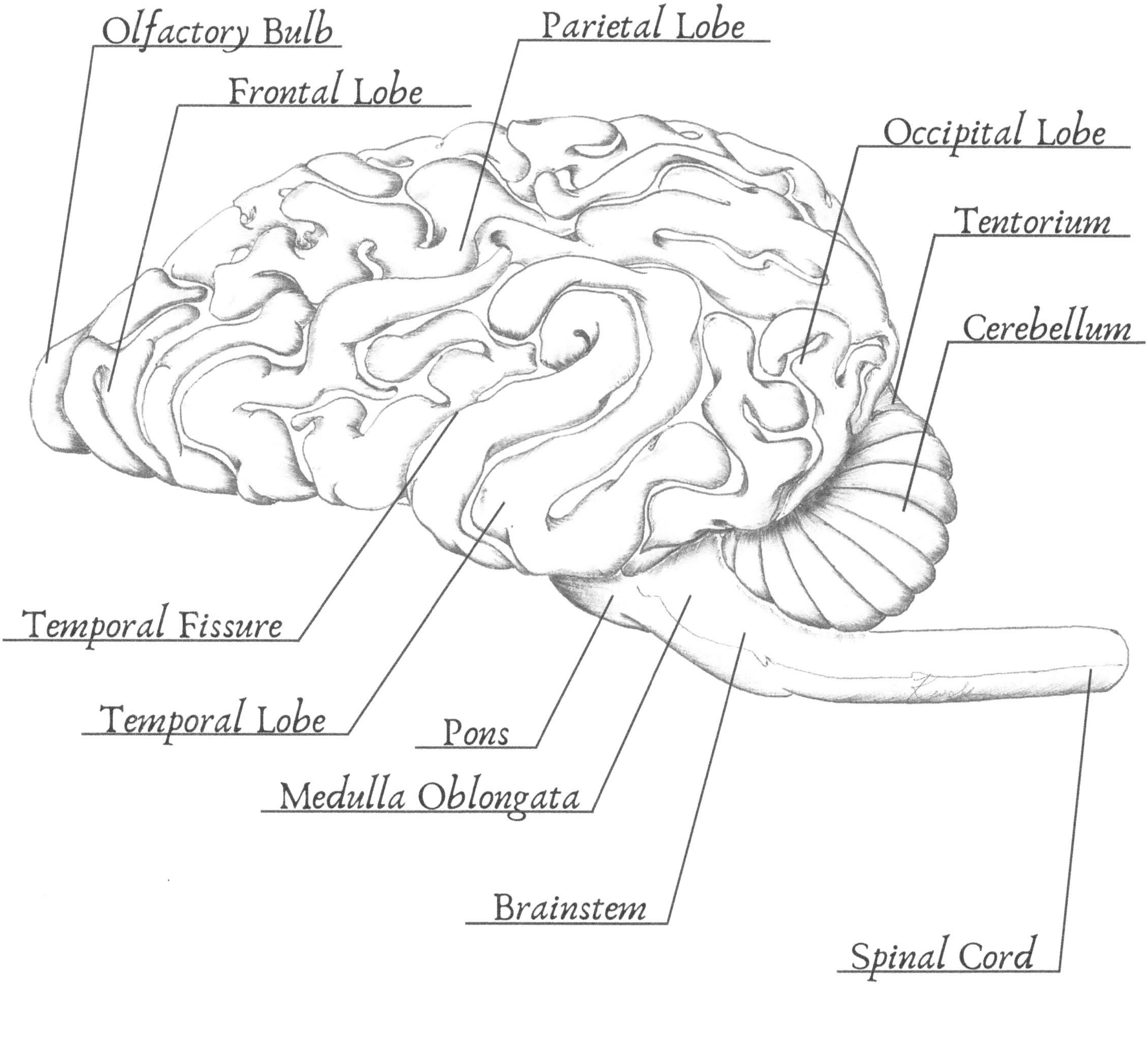

Brain: Lateral View

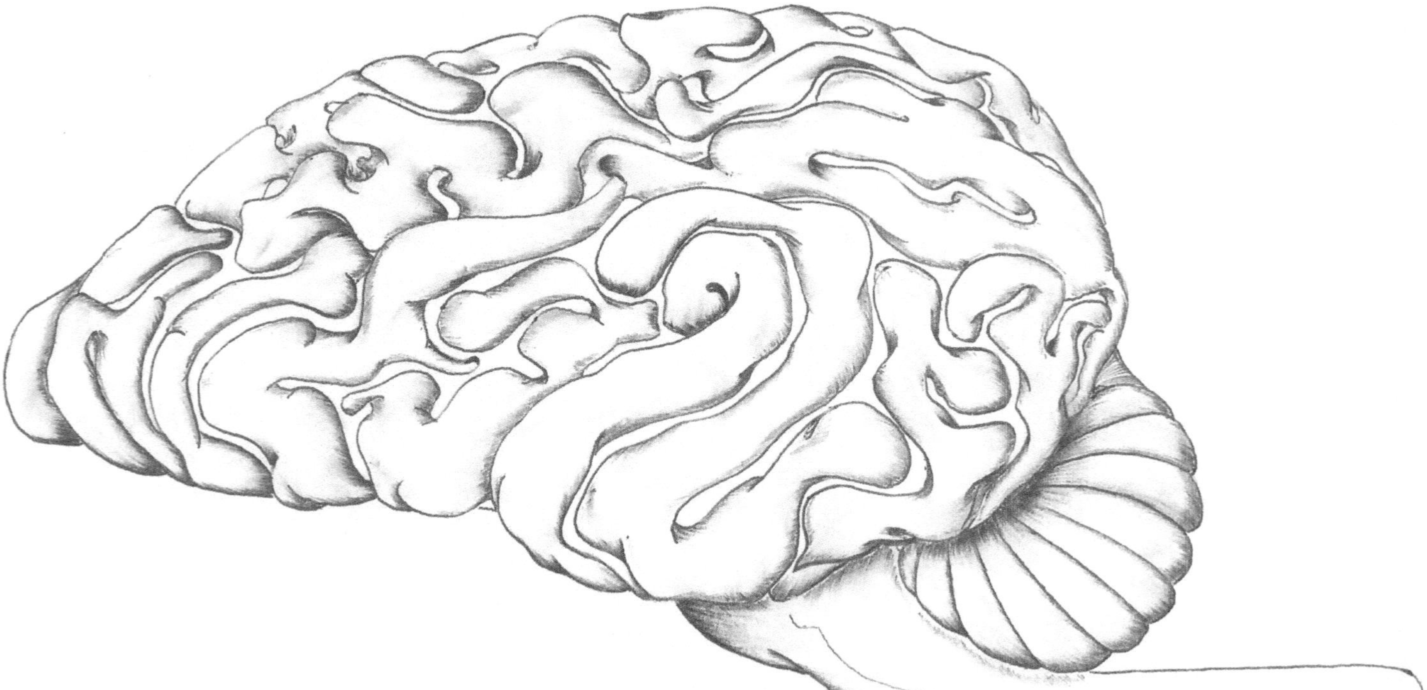

Brain: Mid Sagittal View

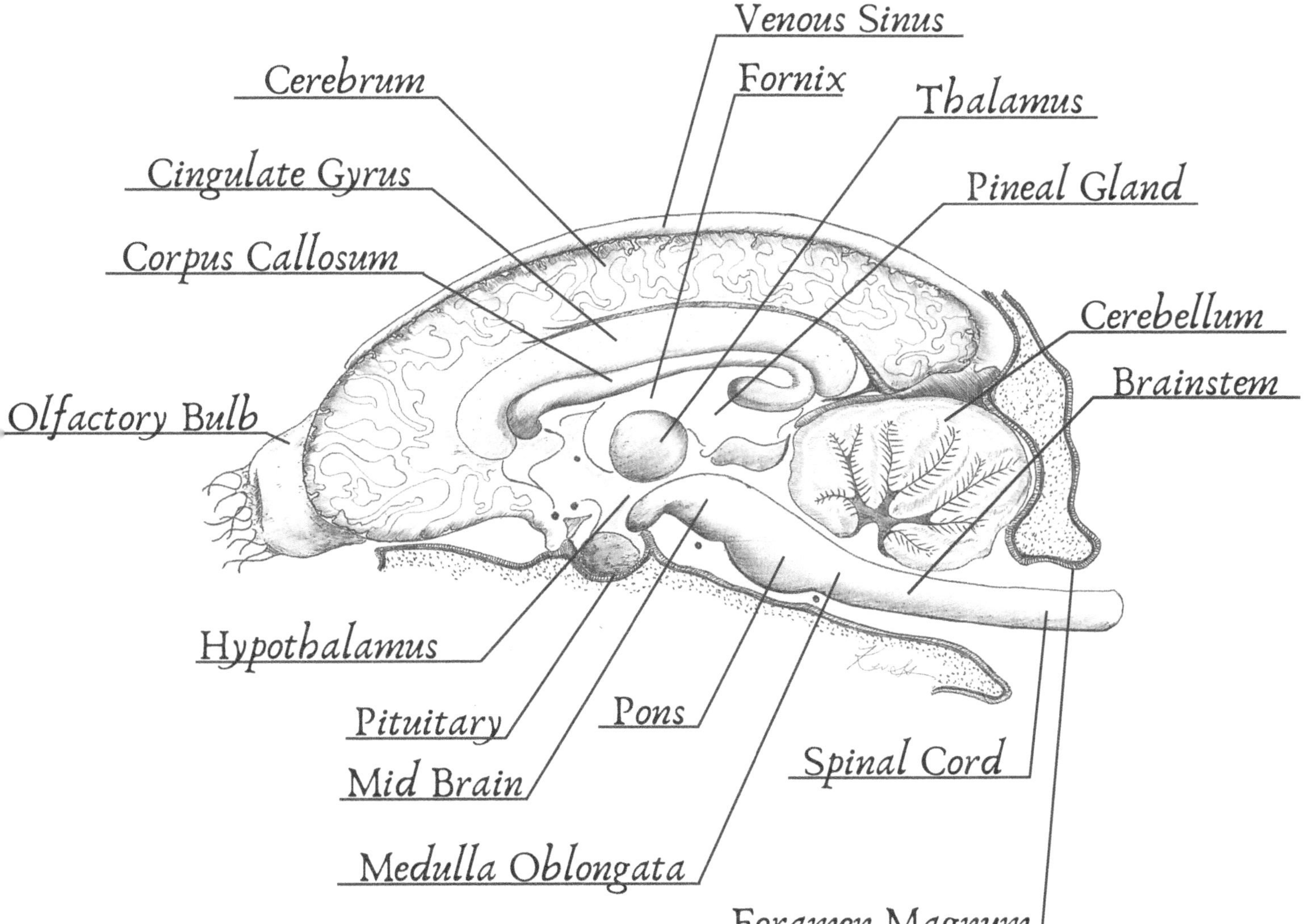

Brain: Mid Sagittal View

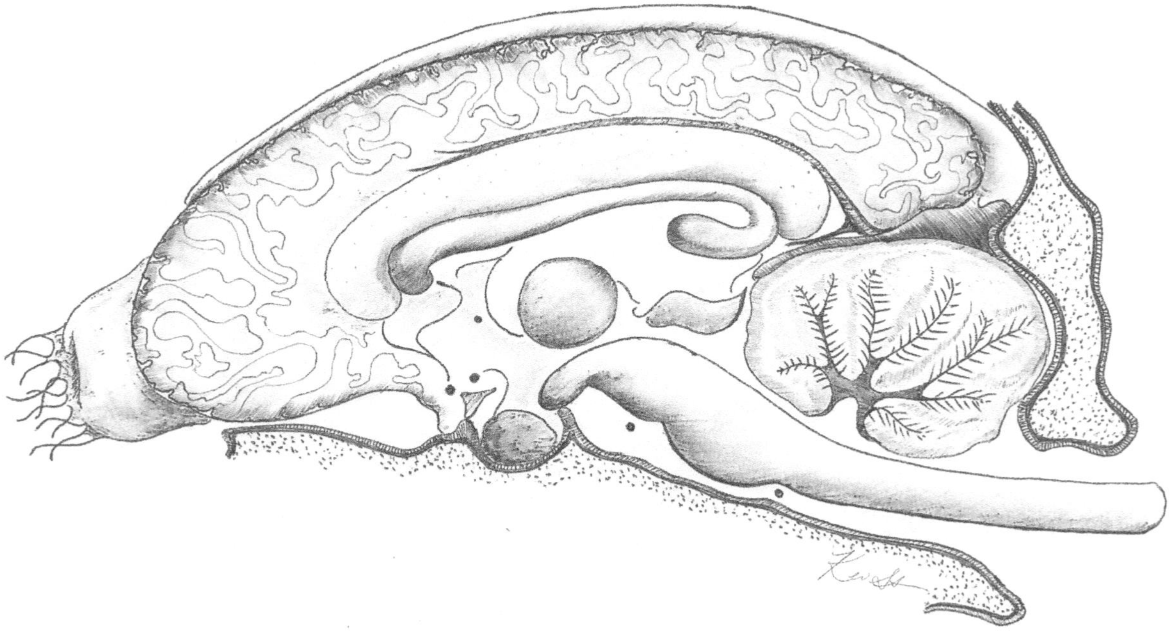

Circle of Willis: Inferior View

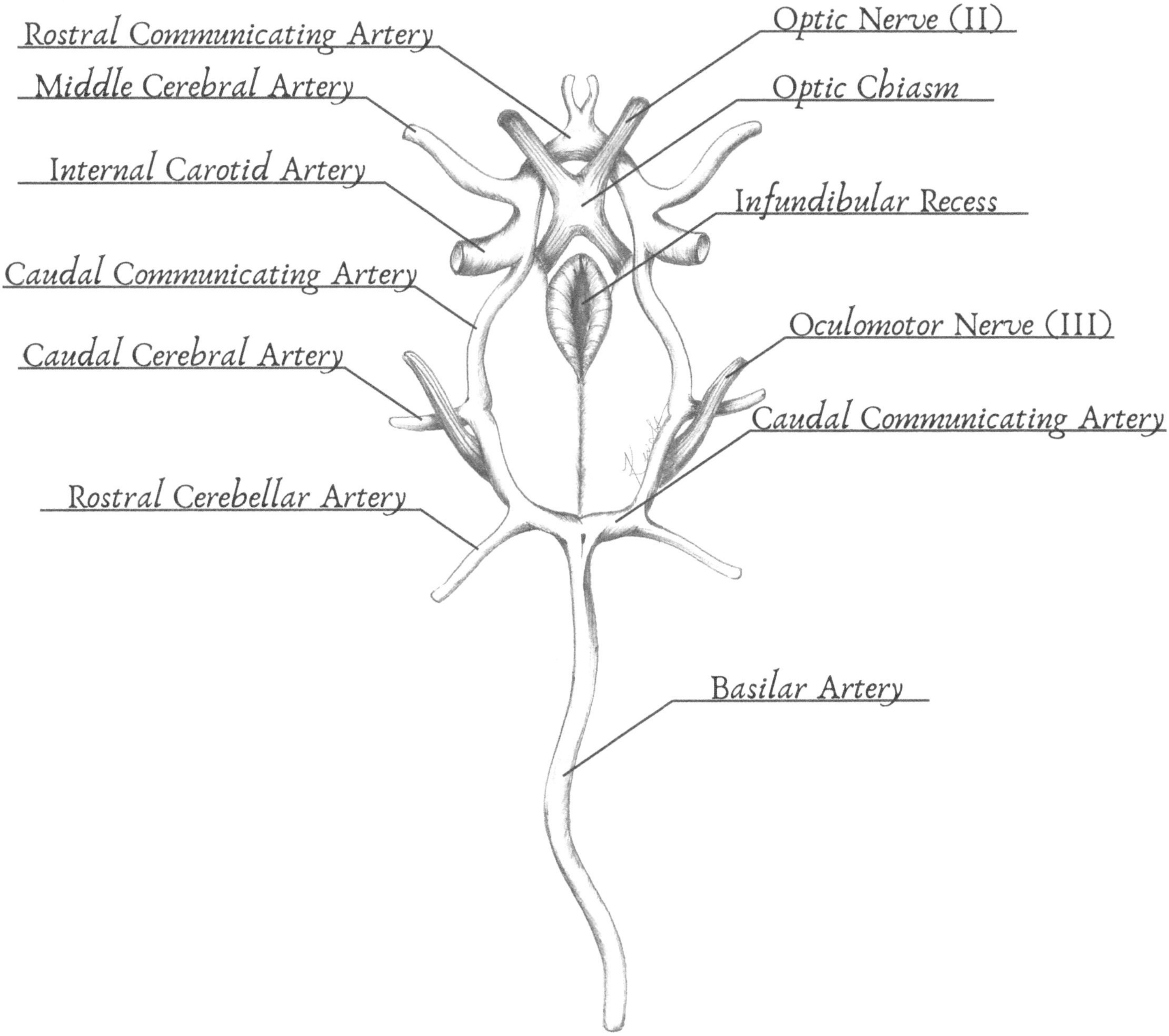

Circle of Willis: Inferior View

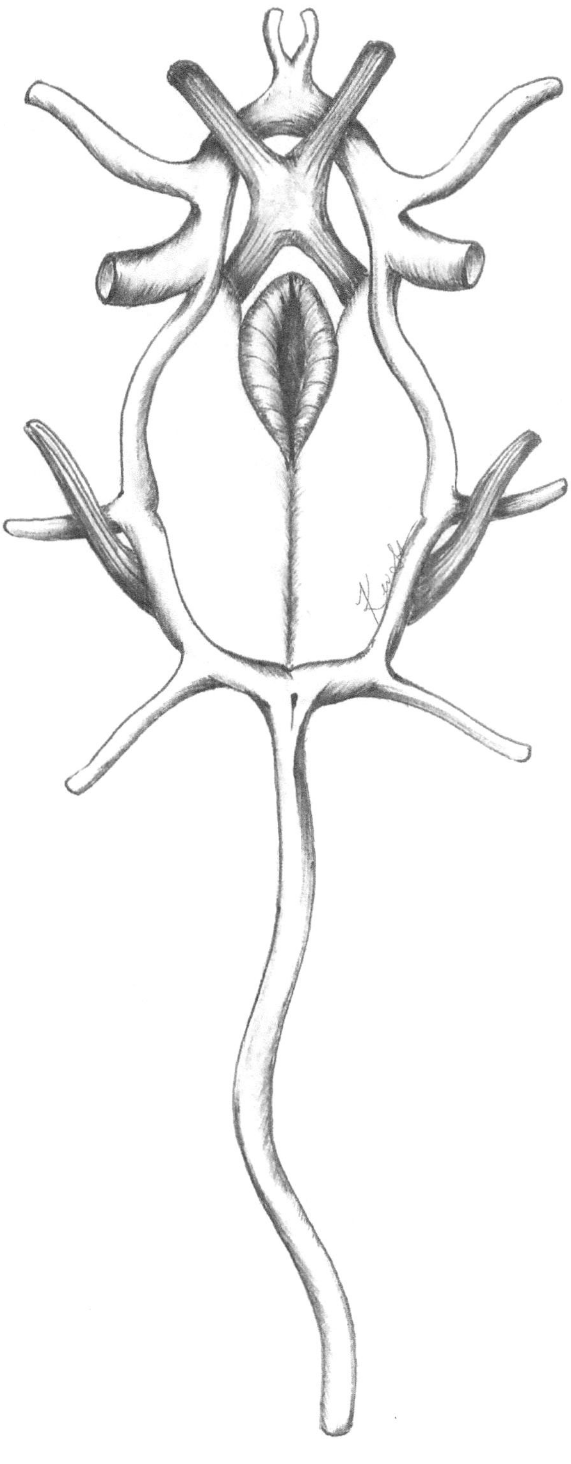

Cranial Nerves: Inferior View

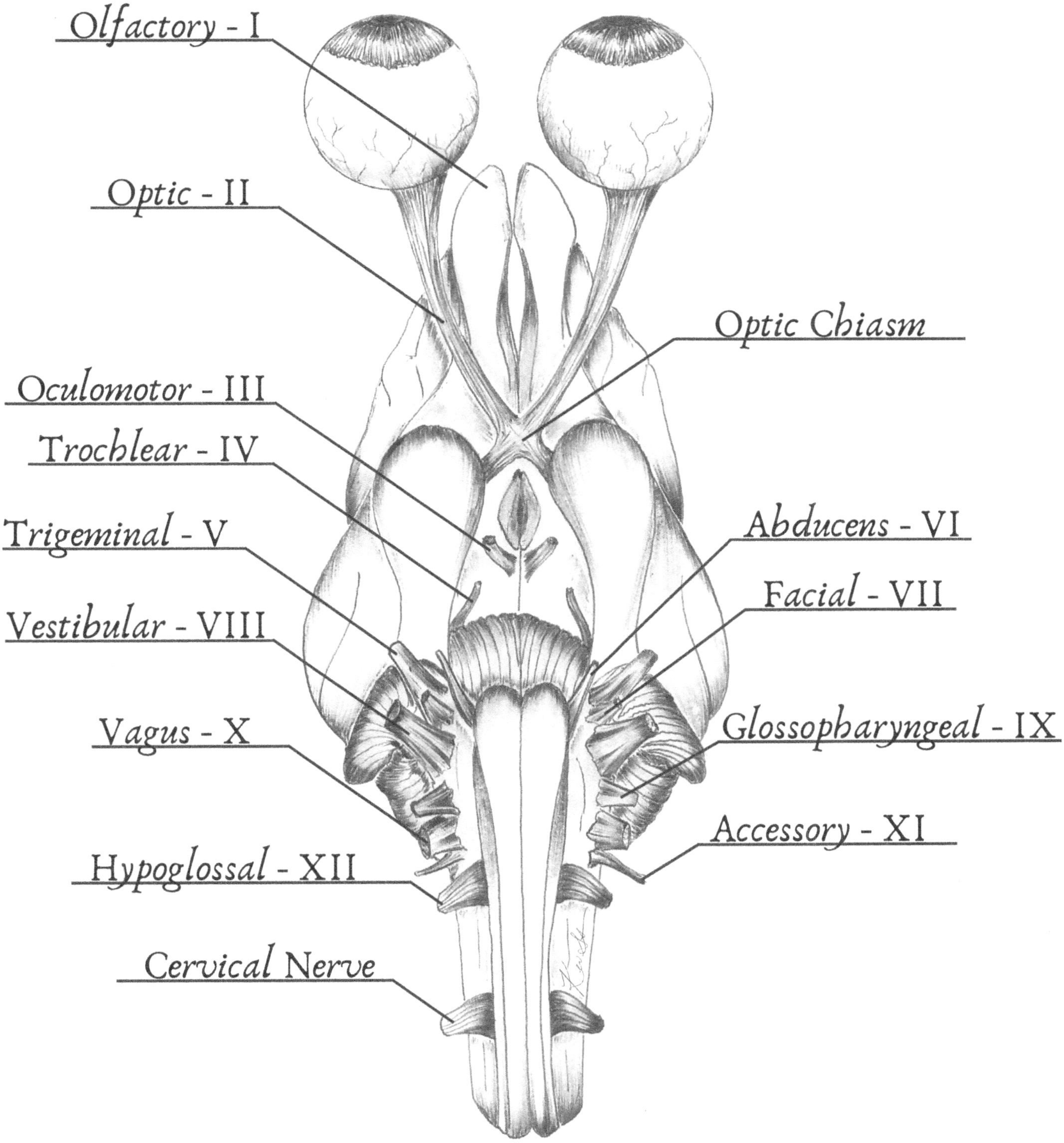

Cranial Nerves: Inferior View

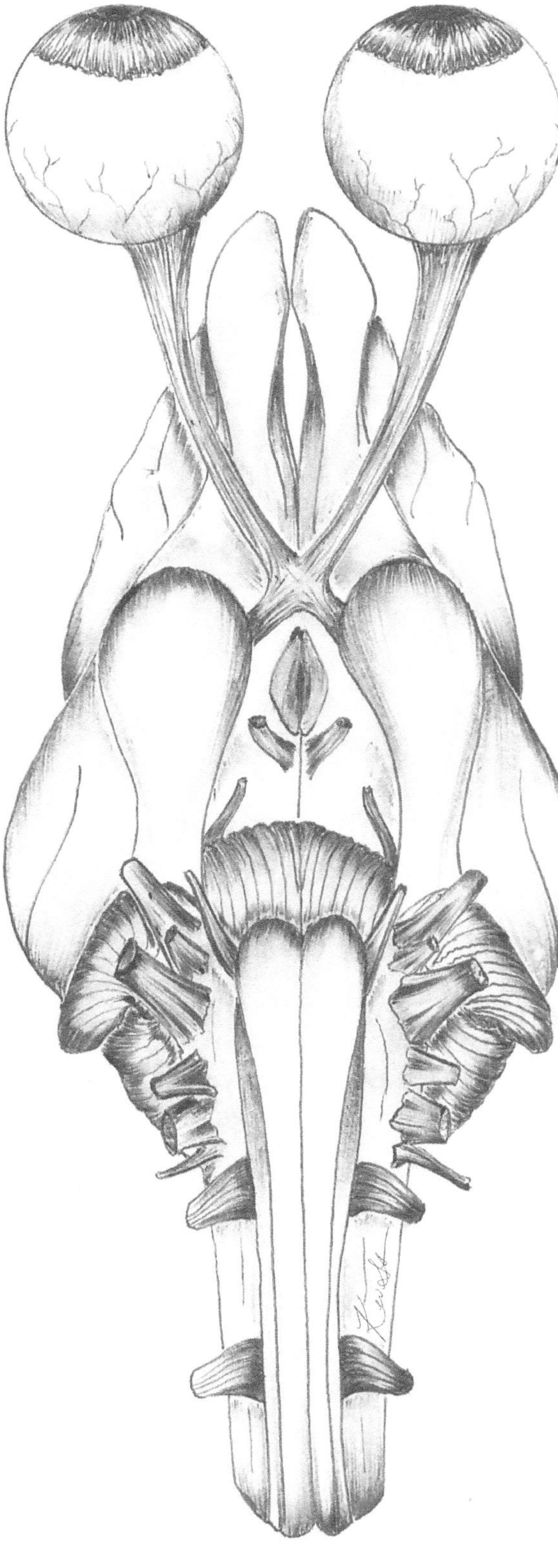

the Eye: Anterior View

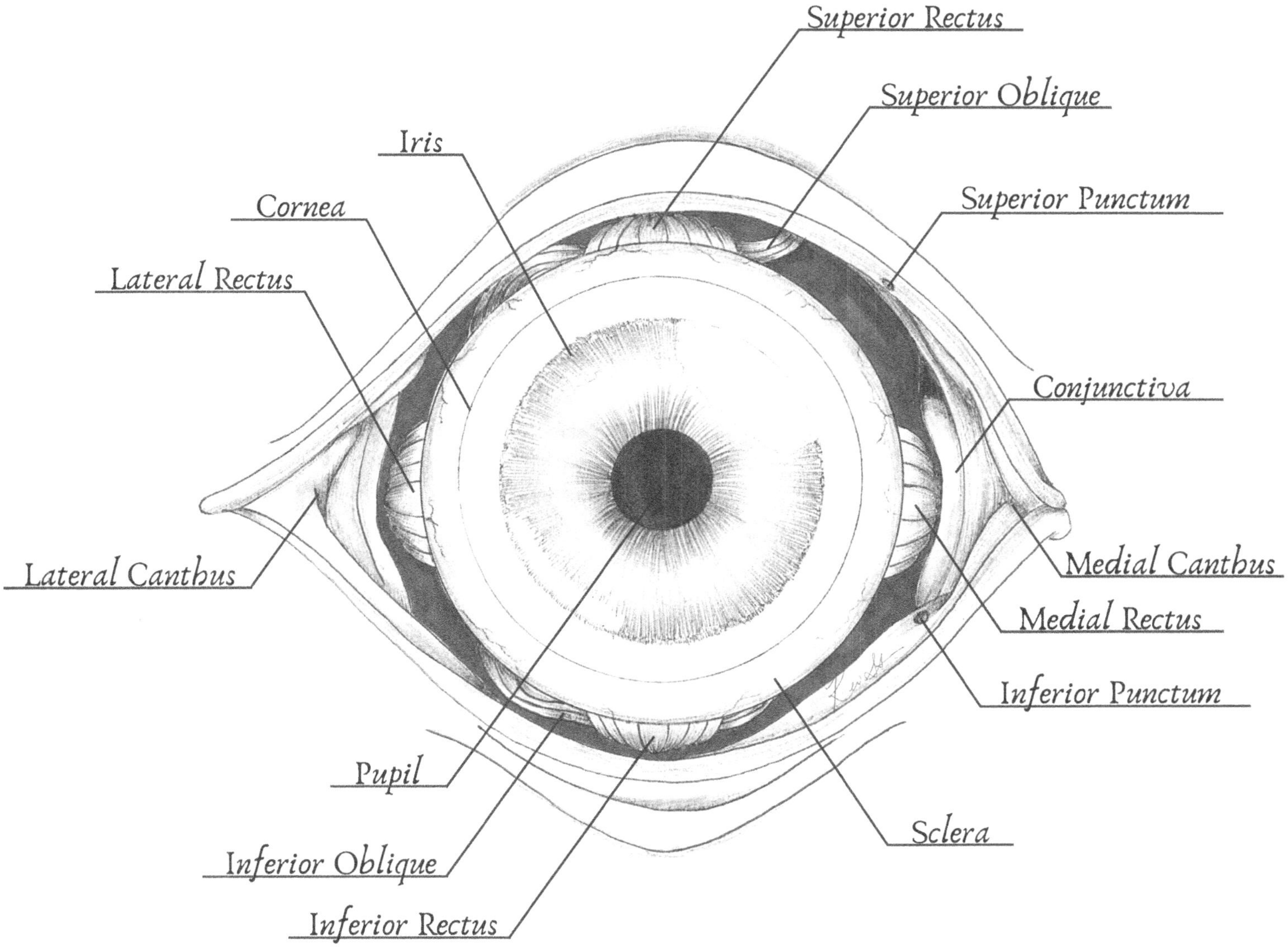

the Eye: Anterior View

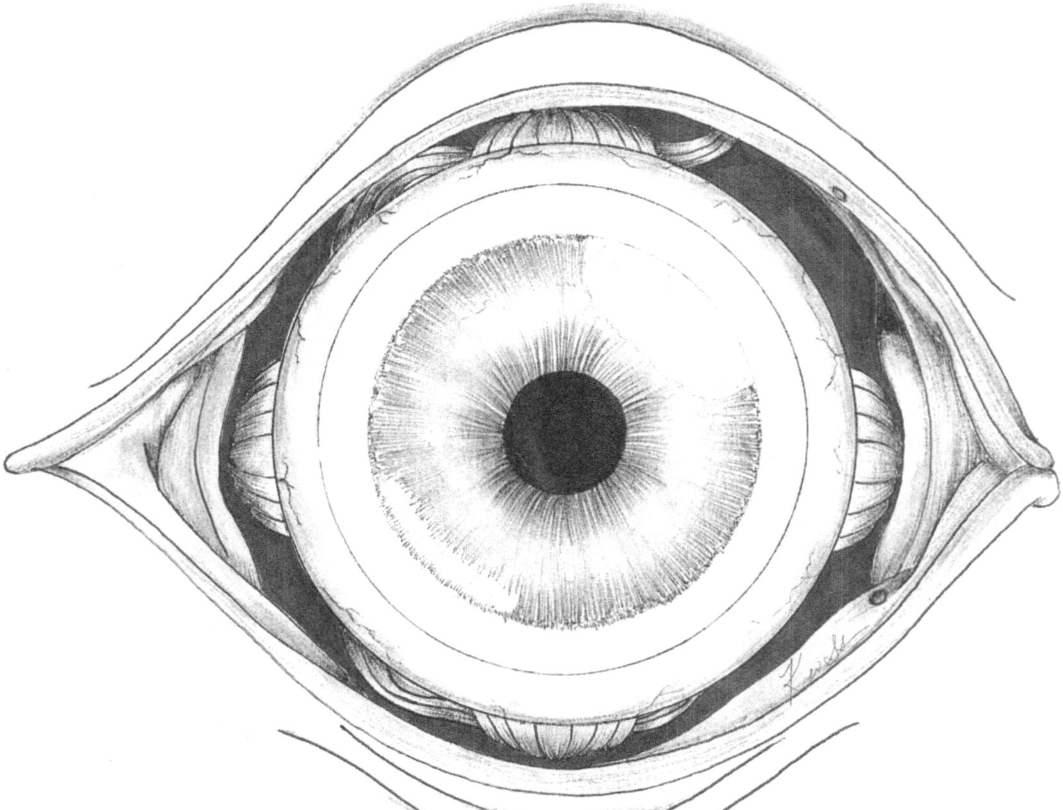

Inner Auditory Canal: Anterior View

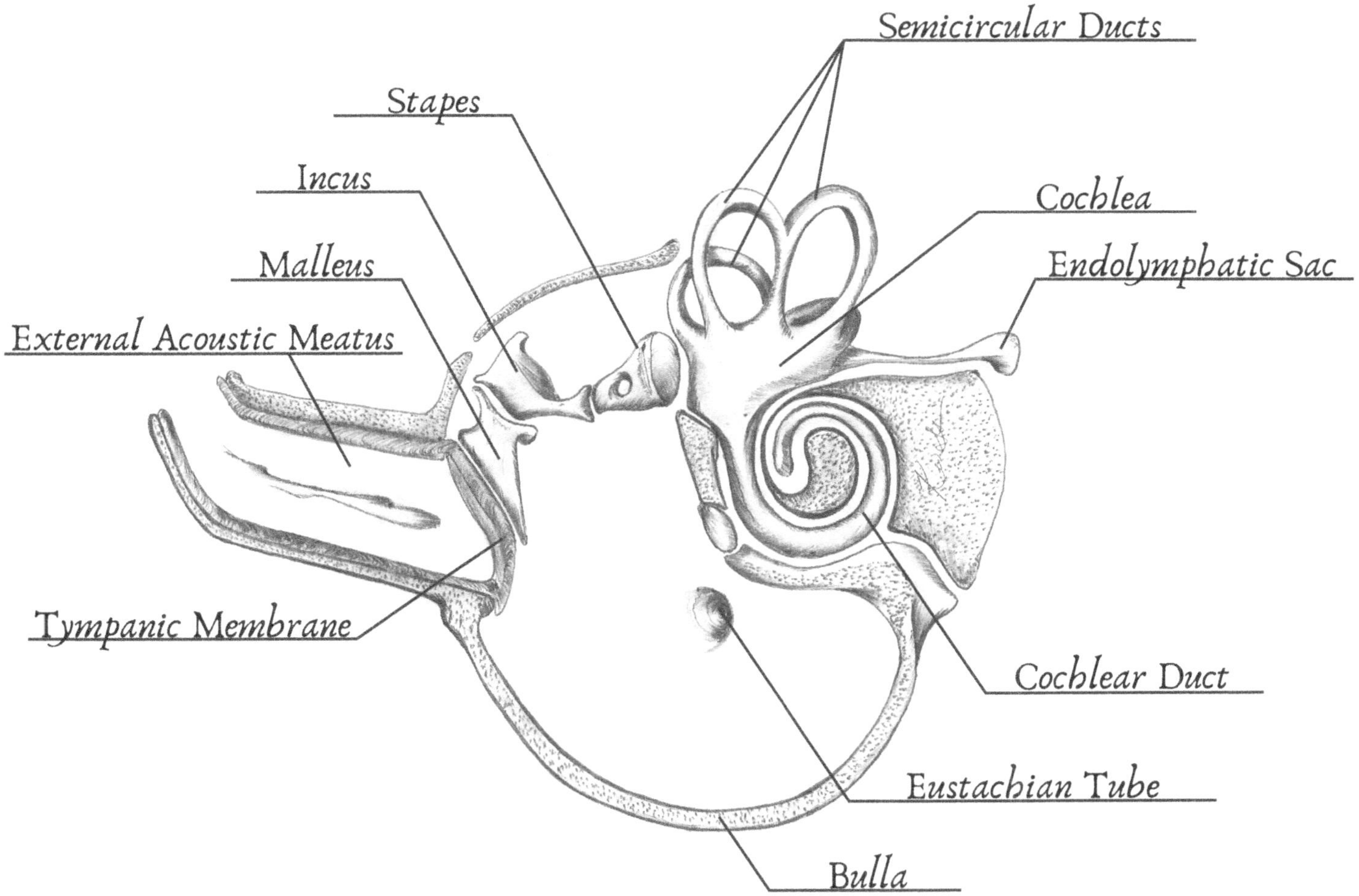

Inner Auditory Canal: Anterior View

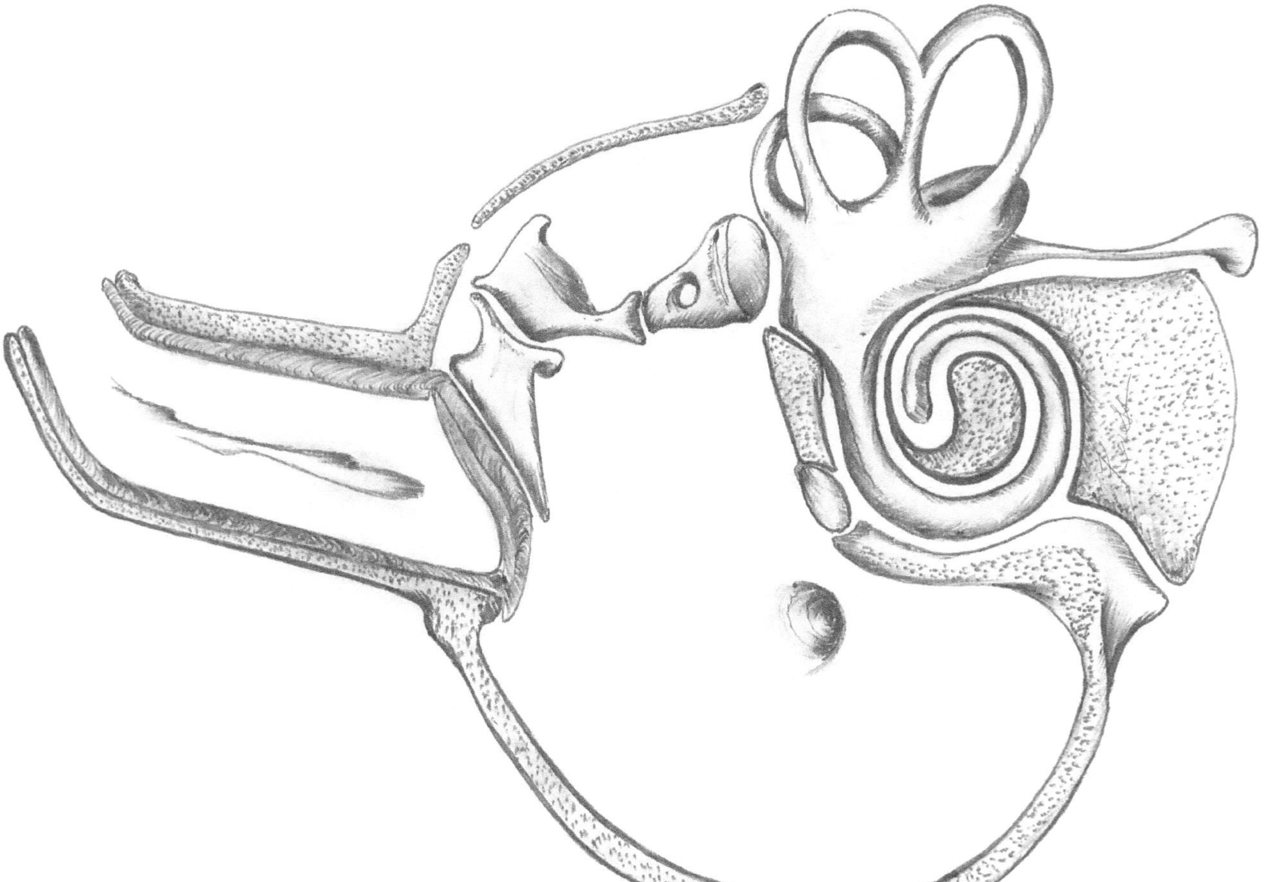

the Neuron

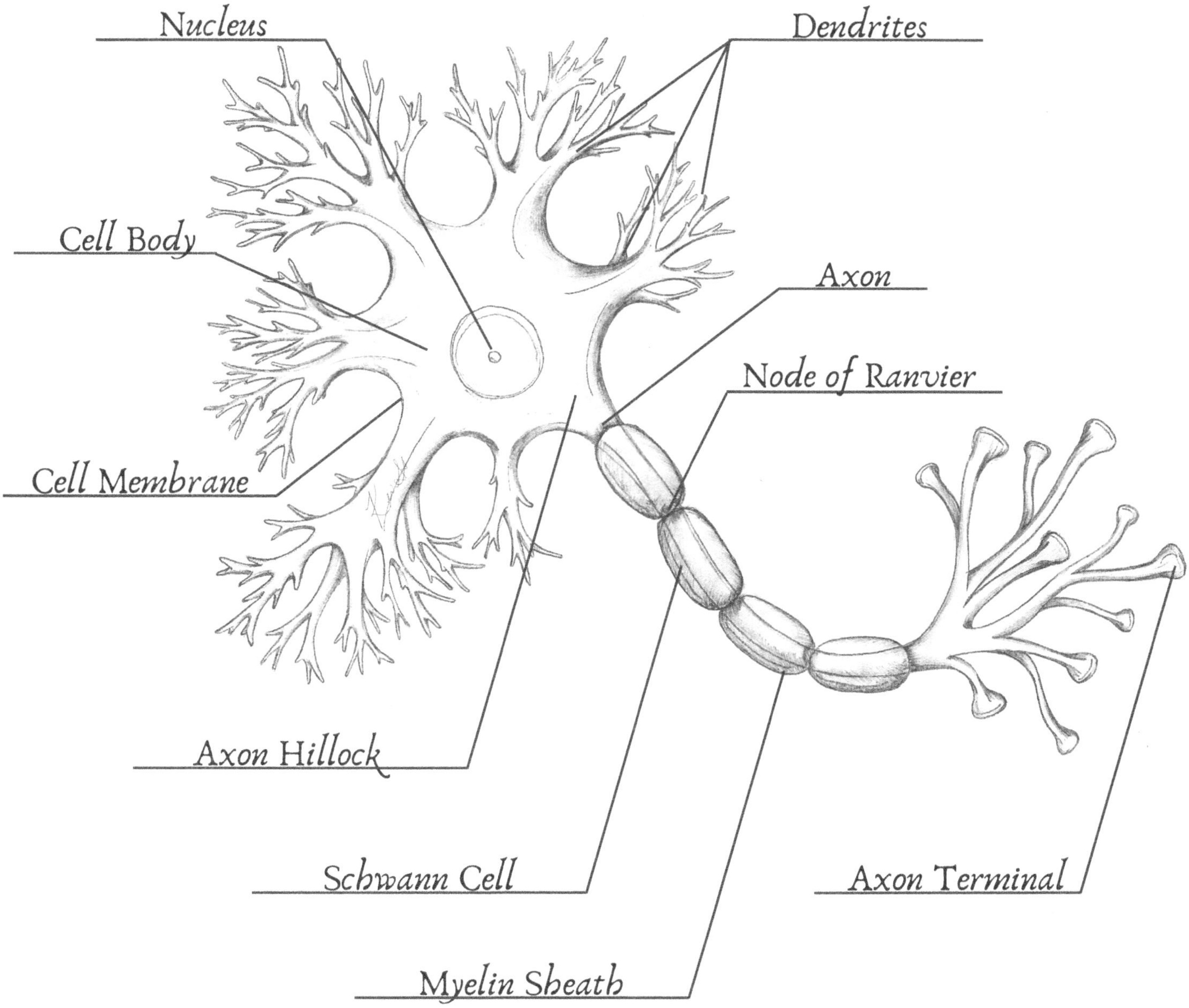

Nucleus
Dendrites
Cell Body
Axon
Node of Ranvier
Cell Membrane
Axon Hillock
Schwann Cell
Axon Terminal
Myelin Sheath

the Neuron

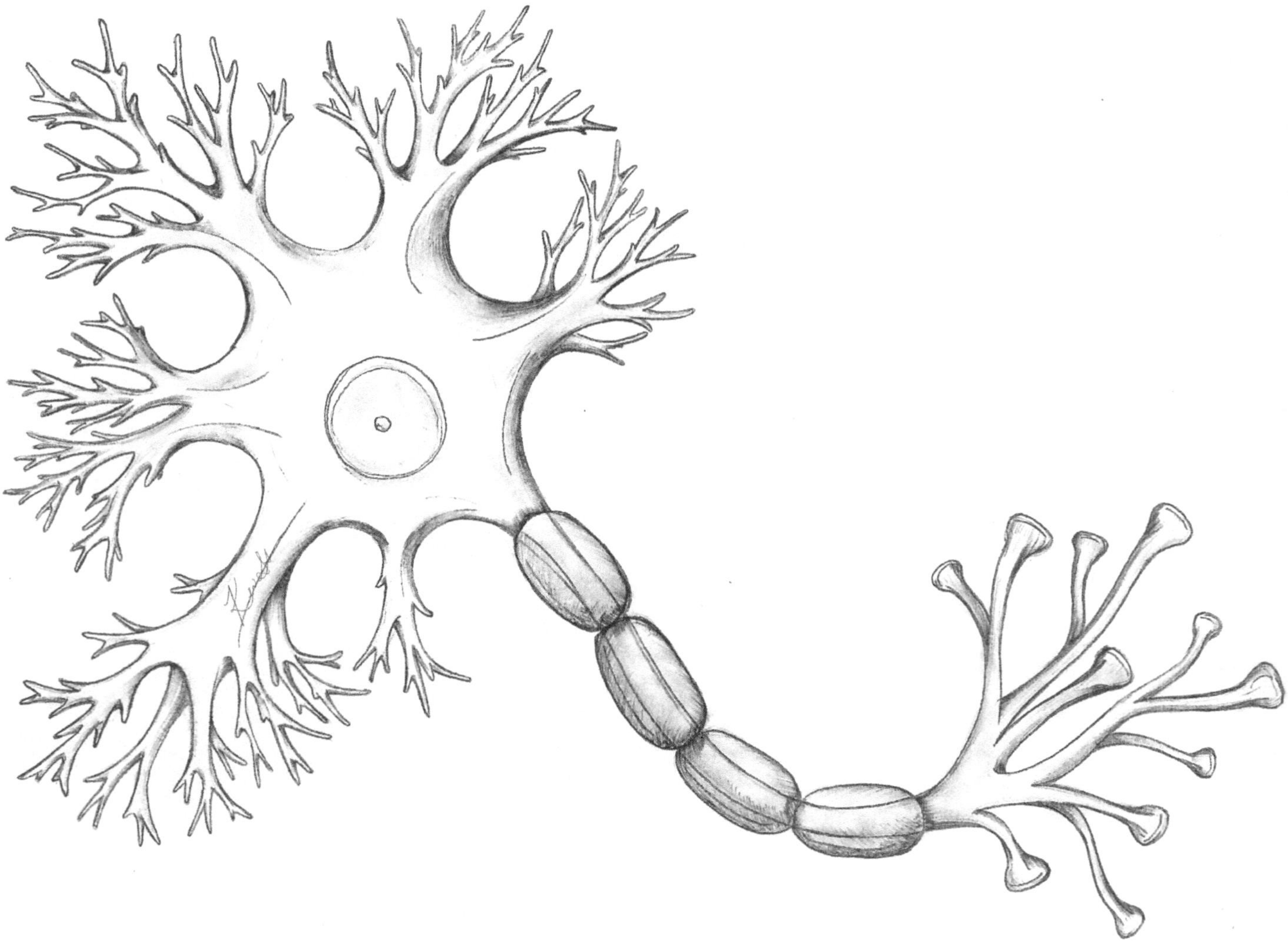

the Spine

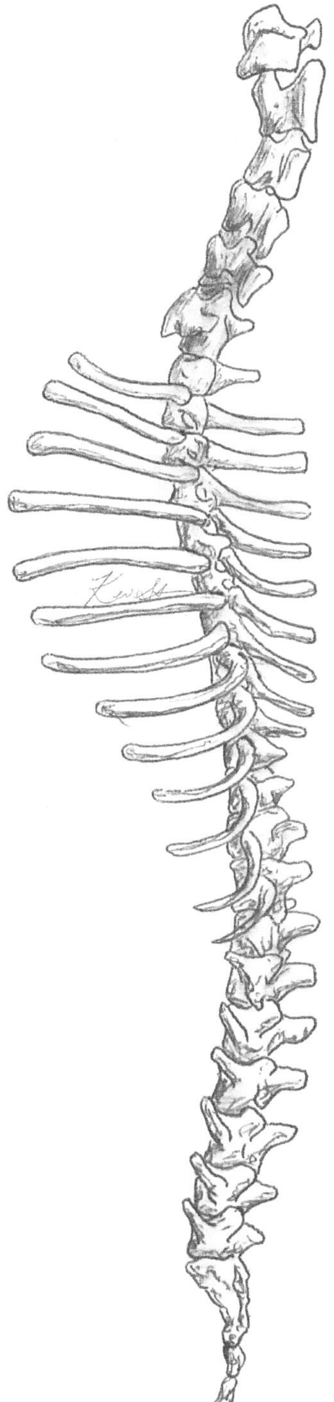

Notes:

- The spine serves to protect the spinal cord and provide skeletal structure.
- The spinal vertebrae include, 7 Cervical, 13 Thoracic, 7 Lumbar, 3 Sacral, as well as 20+ Coccygeal vertebrae.
- Some dogs may have 14 Thoracic or 8 Lumbar vertebrae. This abnormality is more common in certain breeds such as dachshunds.
- The first and second cervical vertebrae (C1 & C2) are also referred to the Atlas and the Axis.
- T1 (the first thoracic vertebra) is recognized by a longer dorsal spinous process.
- The vertebrae align to each other at their articular facets.
- A round opening, called the foramen between the vertebrae provides an exit for nerves branching off of the spinal cord.
- The brachial plexus is a bilaterally symmetrical bundle of nerves branching off the spinal cord from C4 to T3 and extending out towards the shoulders.
- Between the vertebrae are intervertebral discs which act as shock absorbers for the spine.
- The intervertebral discs can herniate or rupture causing compression or trauma to the spinal cord.

Complete Spine: Lateral View

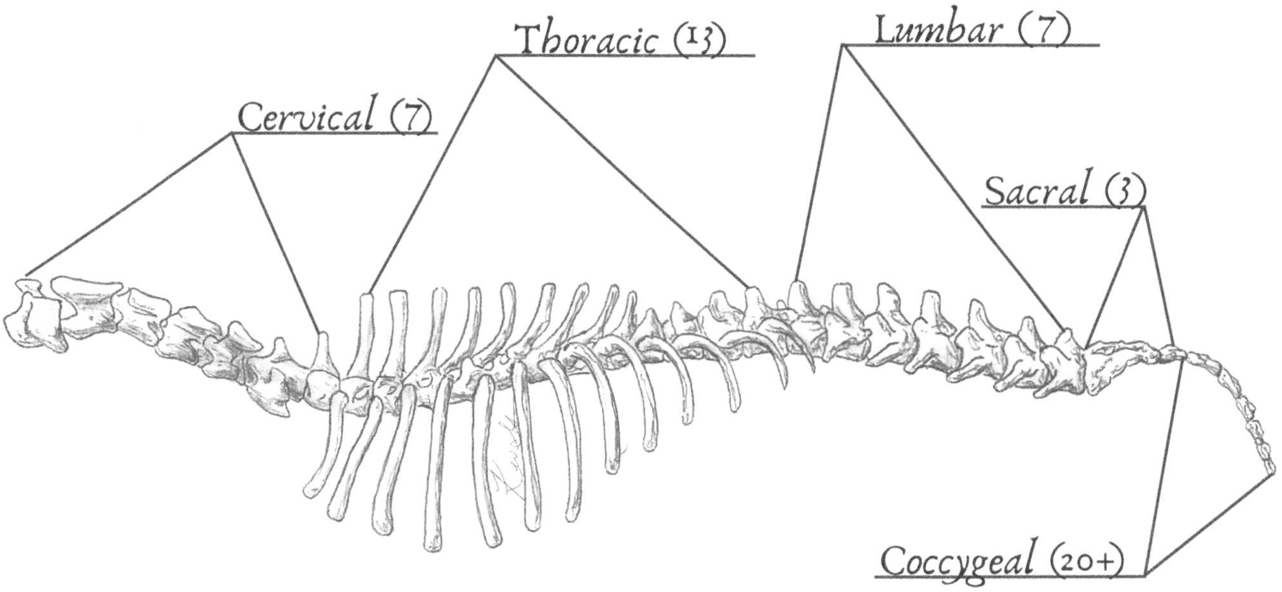

Complete Spine: Lateral View

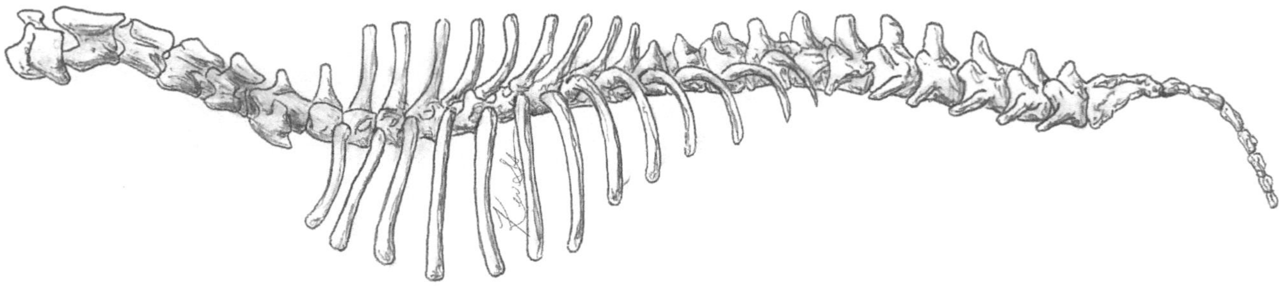

Cervical Spine: Lateral View

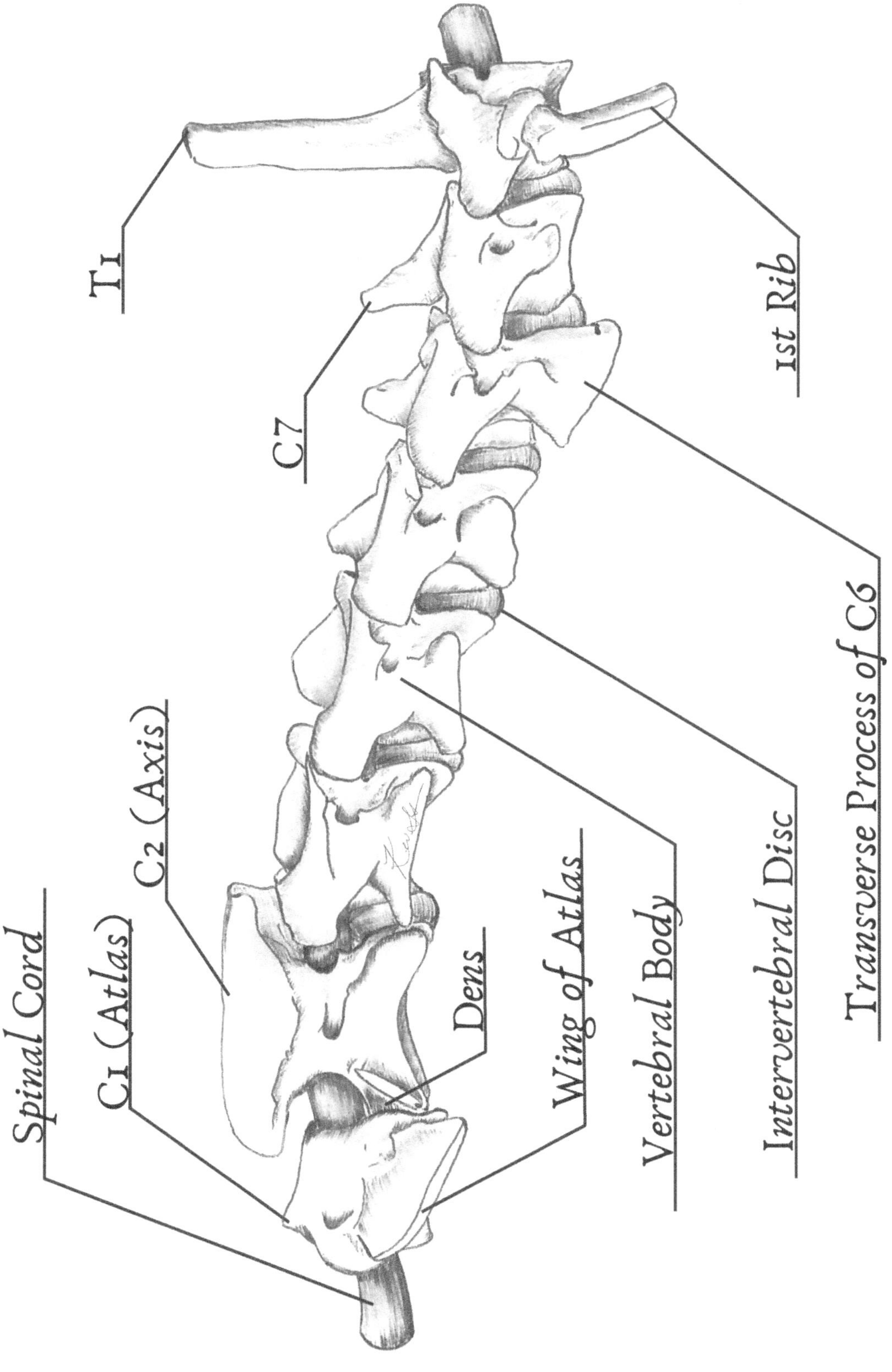

Cervical Spine: Lateral View

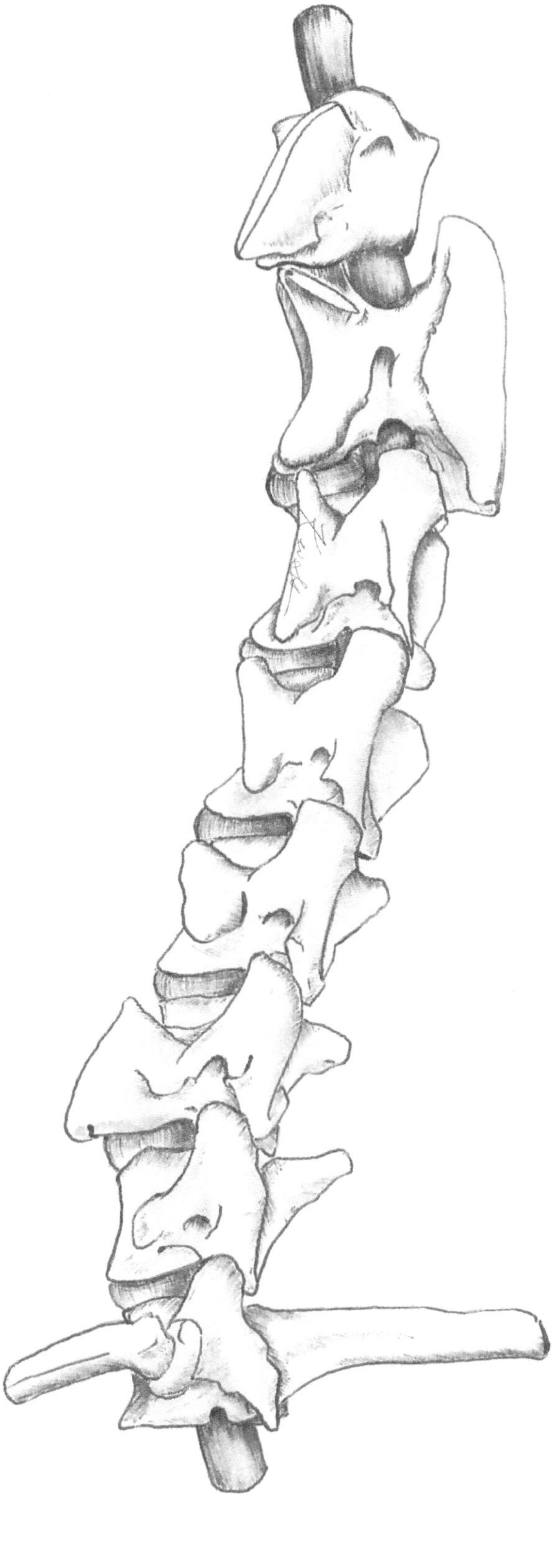

Vertebra: Transverse View

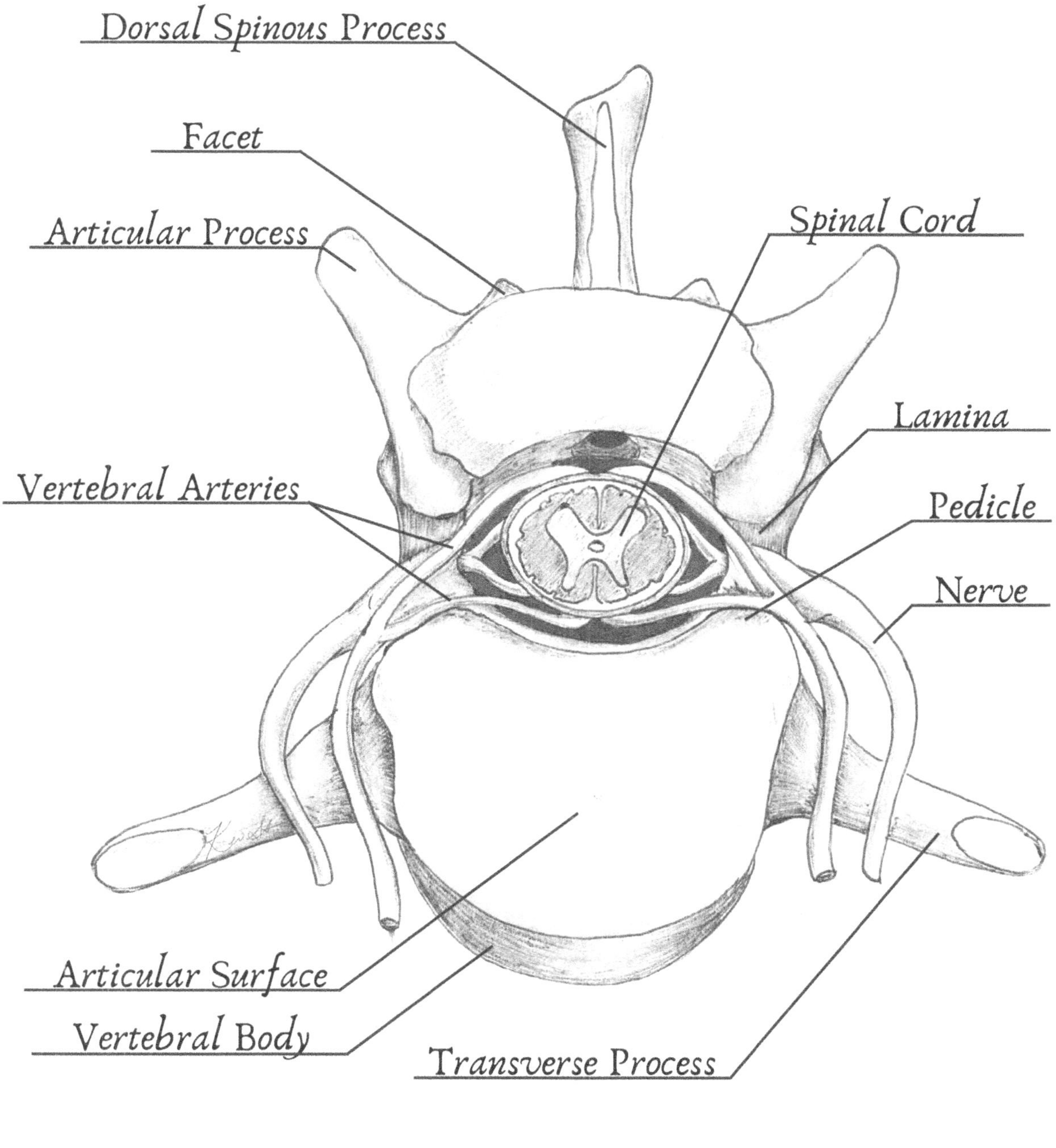

Vertebra: Transverse View

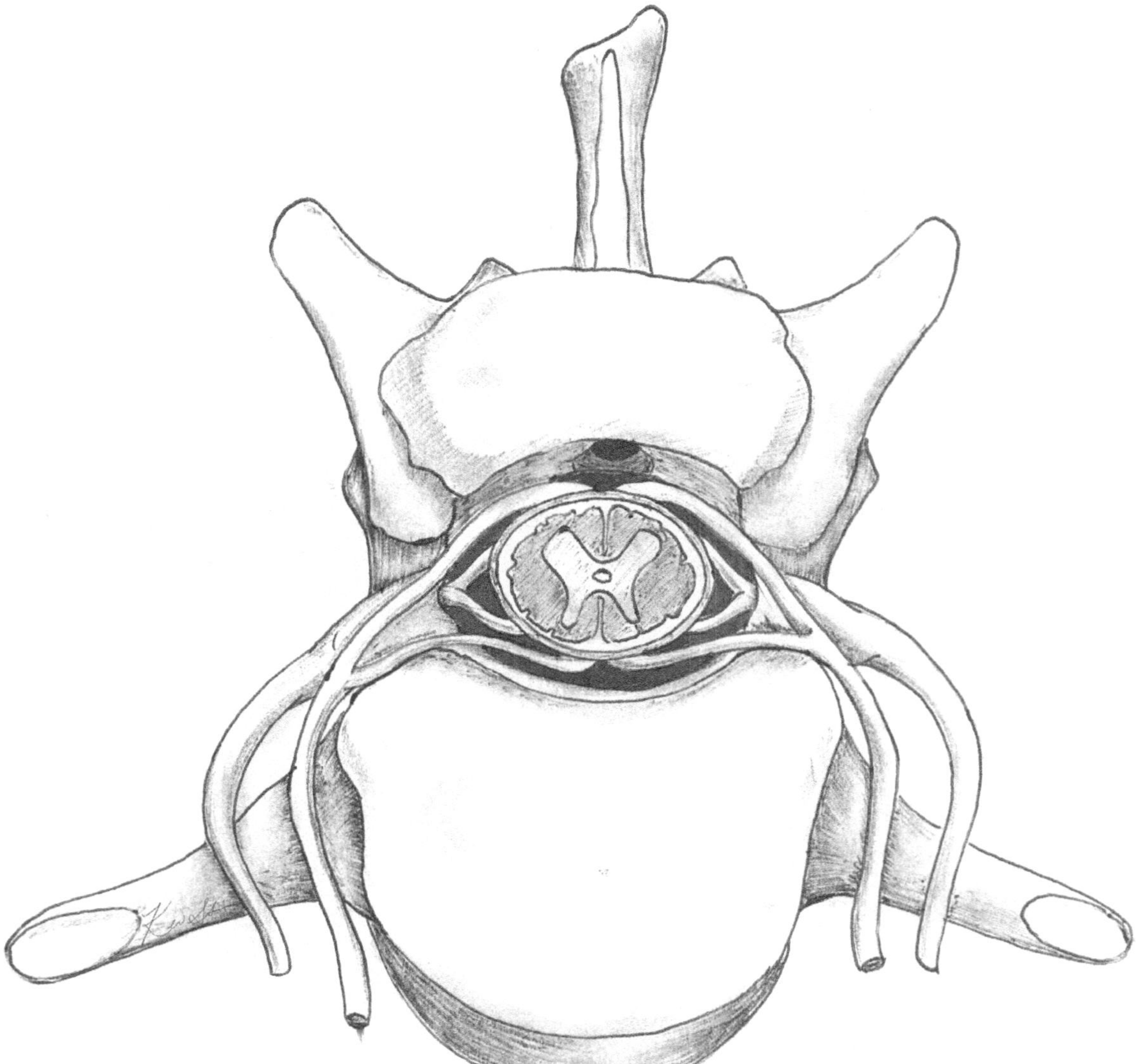

Thoracic Spine: Lateral View

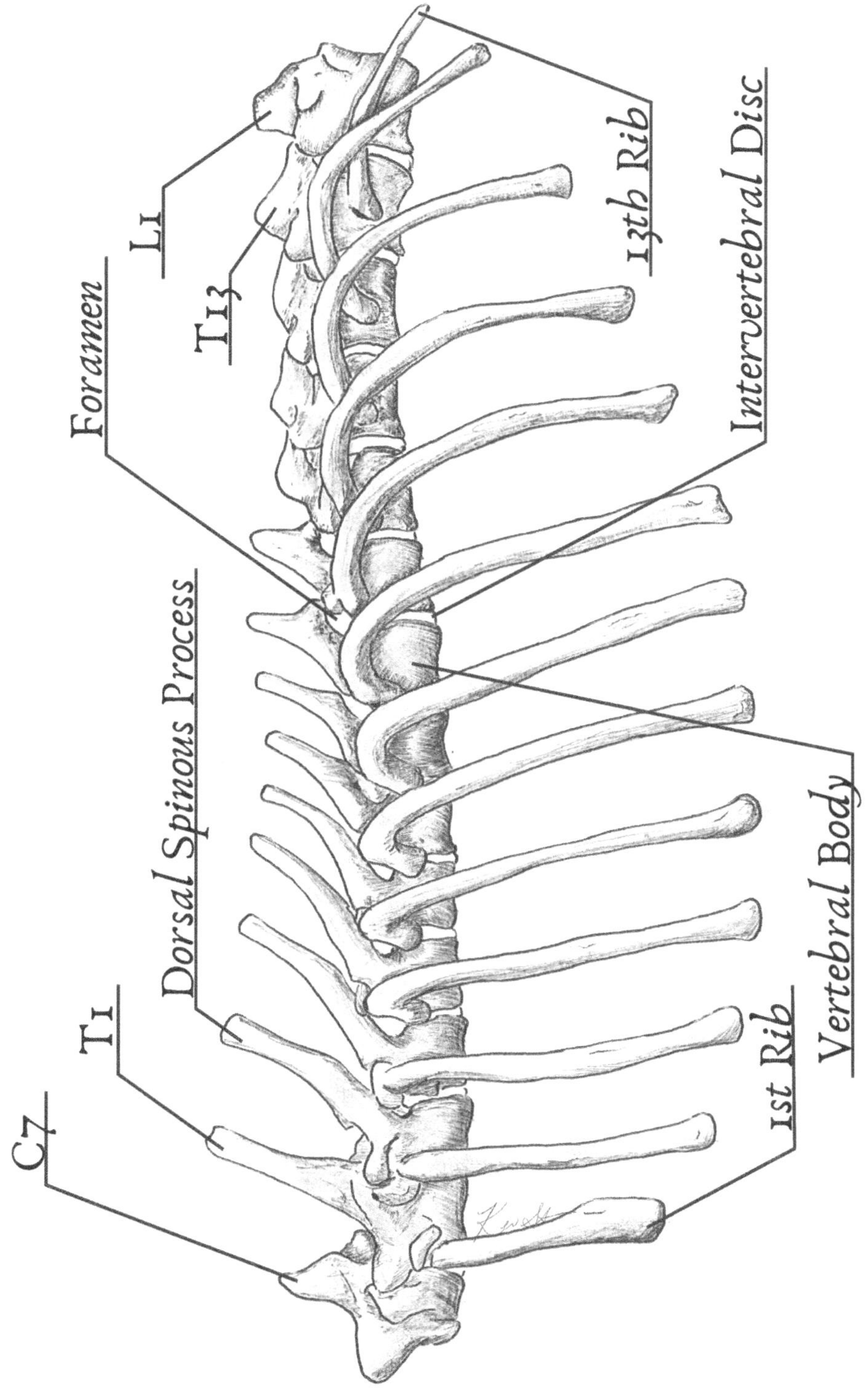

Thoracic Spine

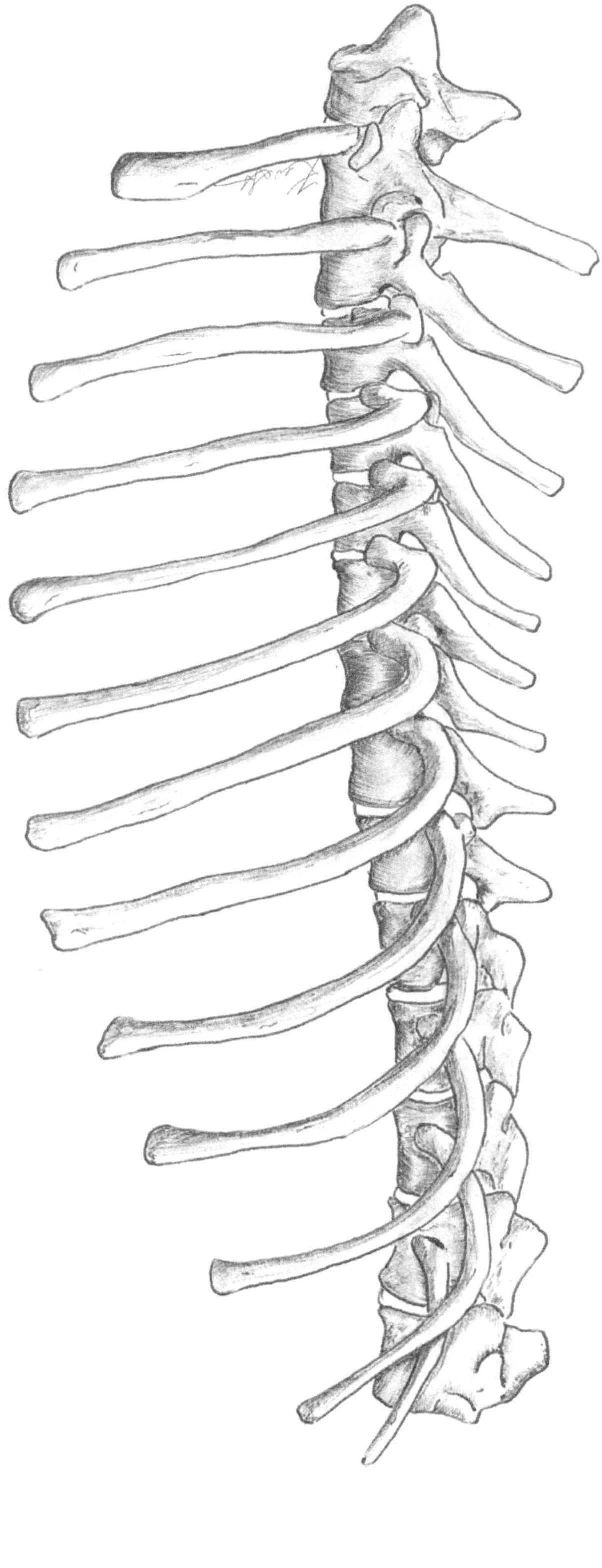

Vertebra

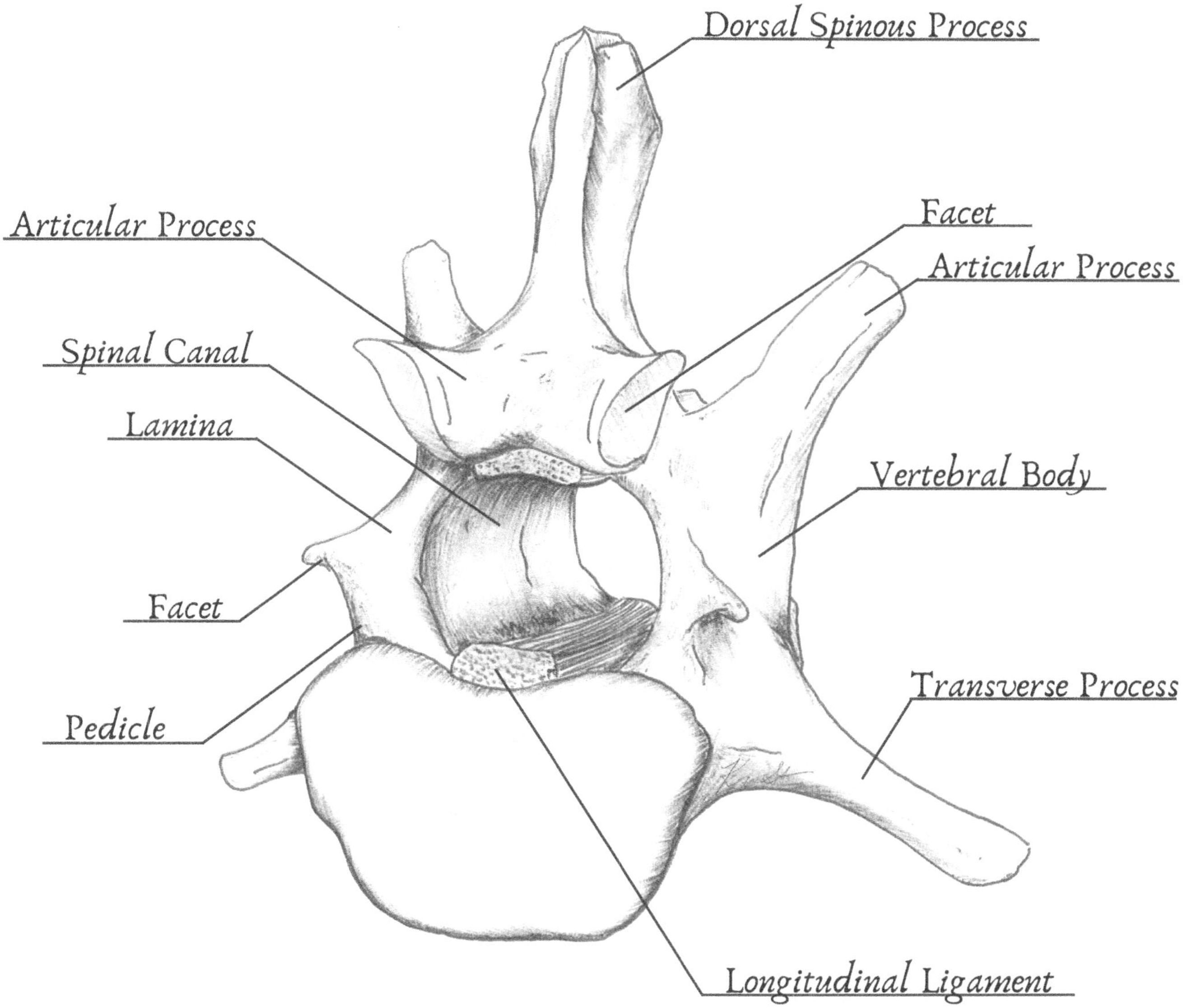
Dorsal Spinous Process
Articular Process
Facet
Articular Process
Spinal Canal
Lamina
Vertebral Body
Facet
Transverse Process
Pedicle
Longitudinal Ligament

Vertebra

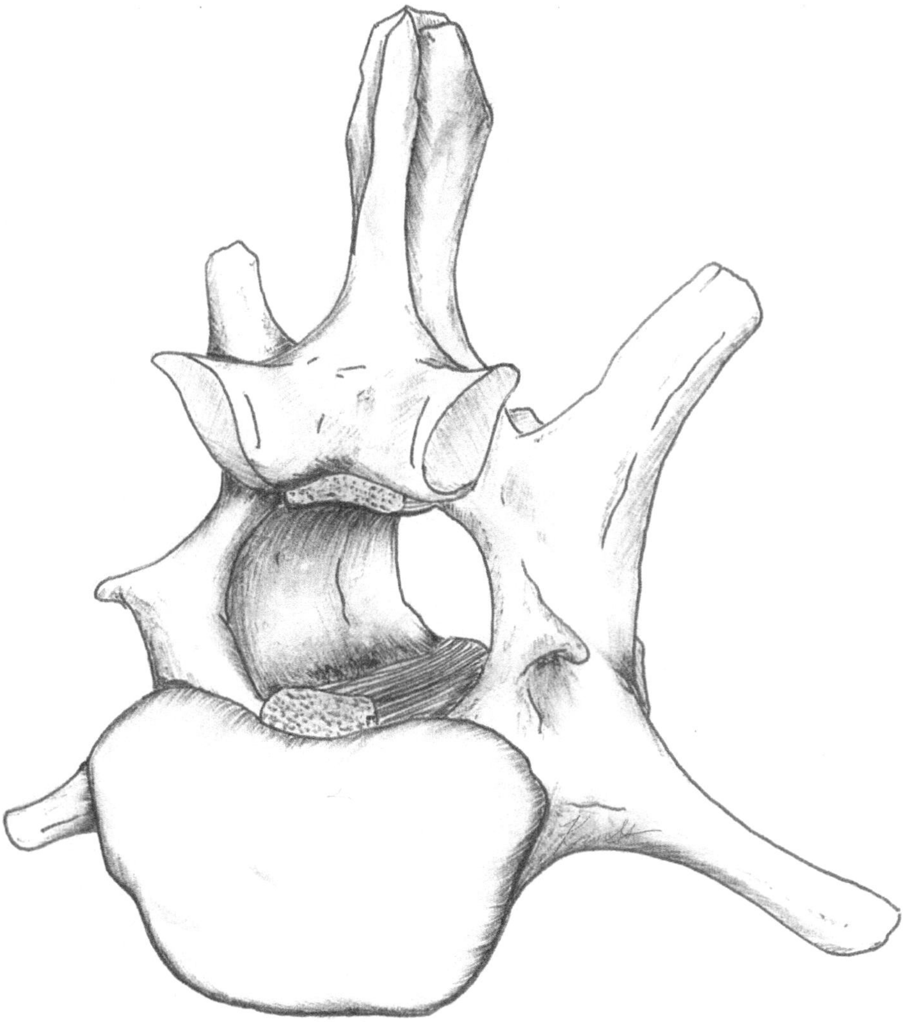

Spinal Cord: Cross Section

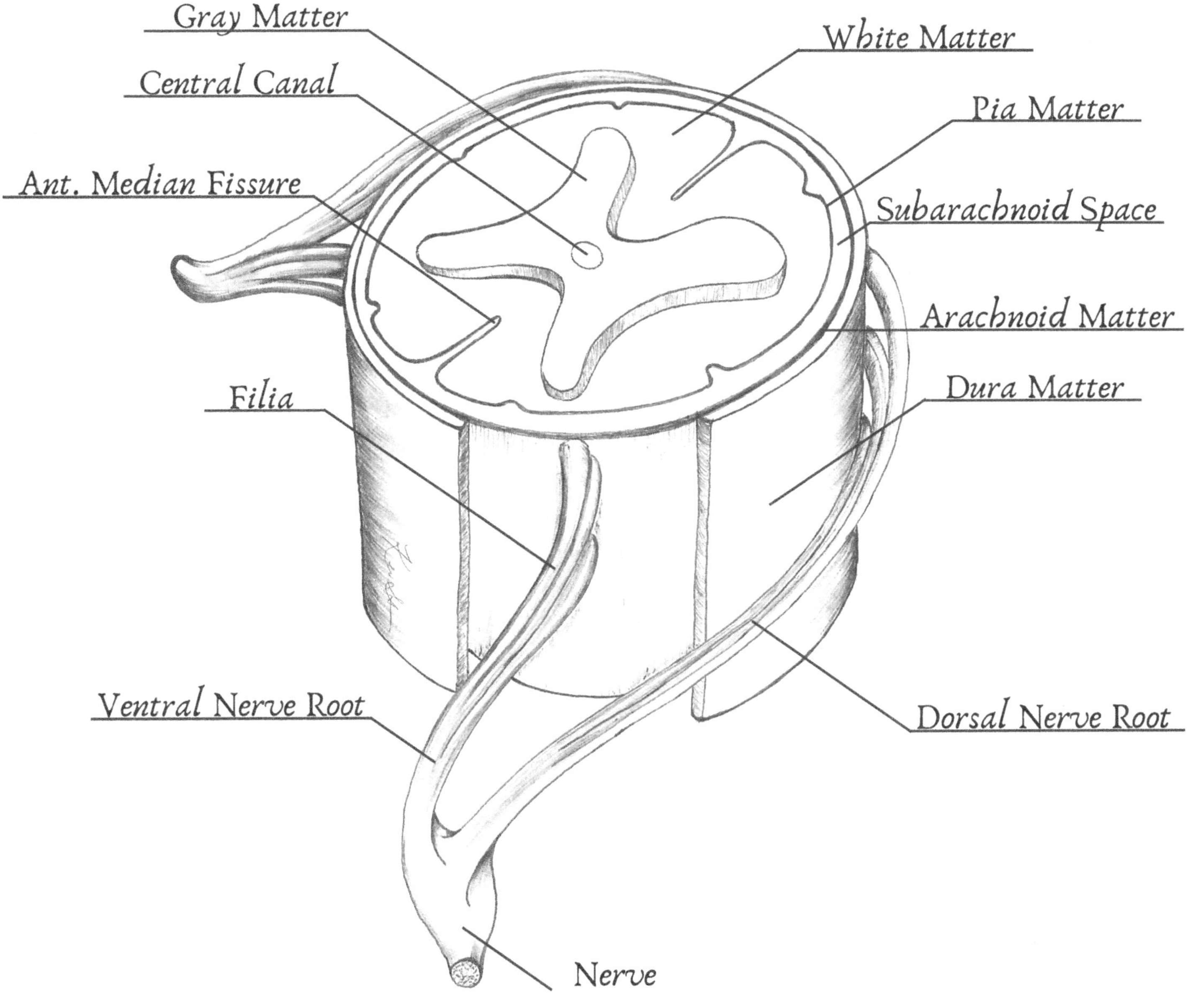

Spinal Cord: Cross Section

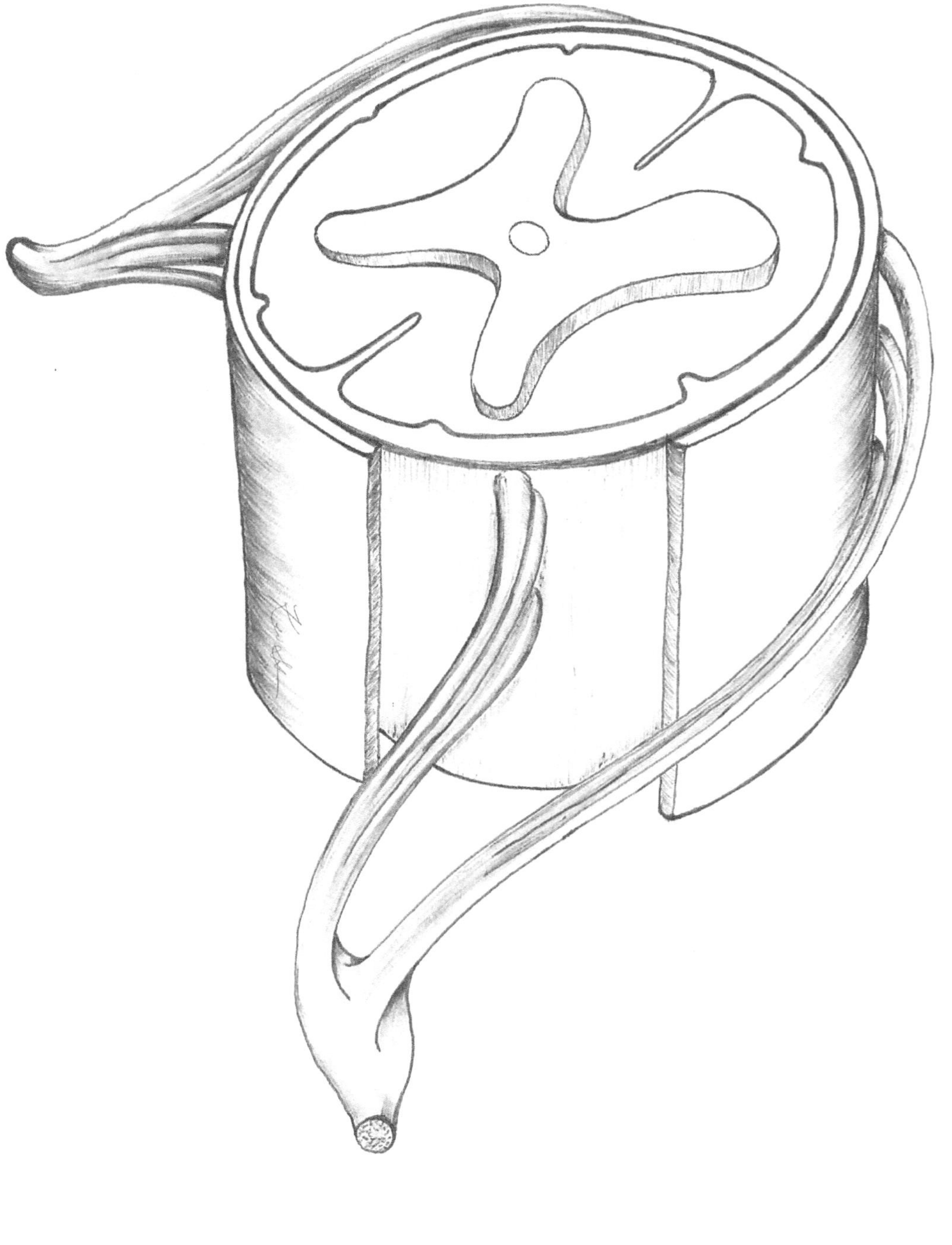

Vertebra: Lateral View

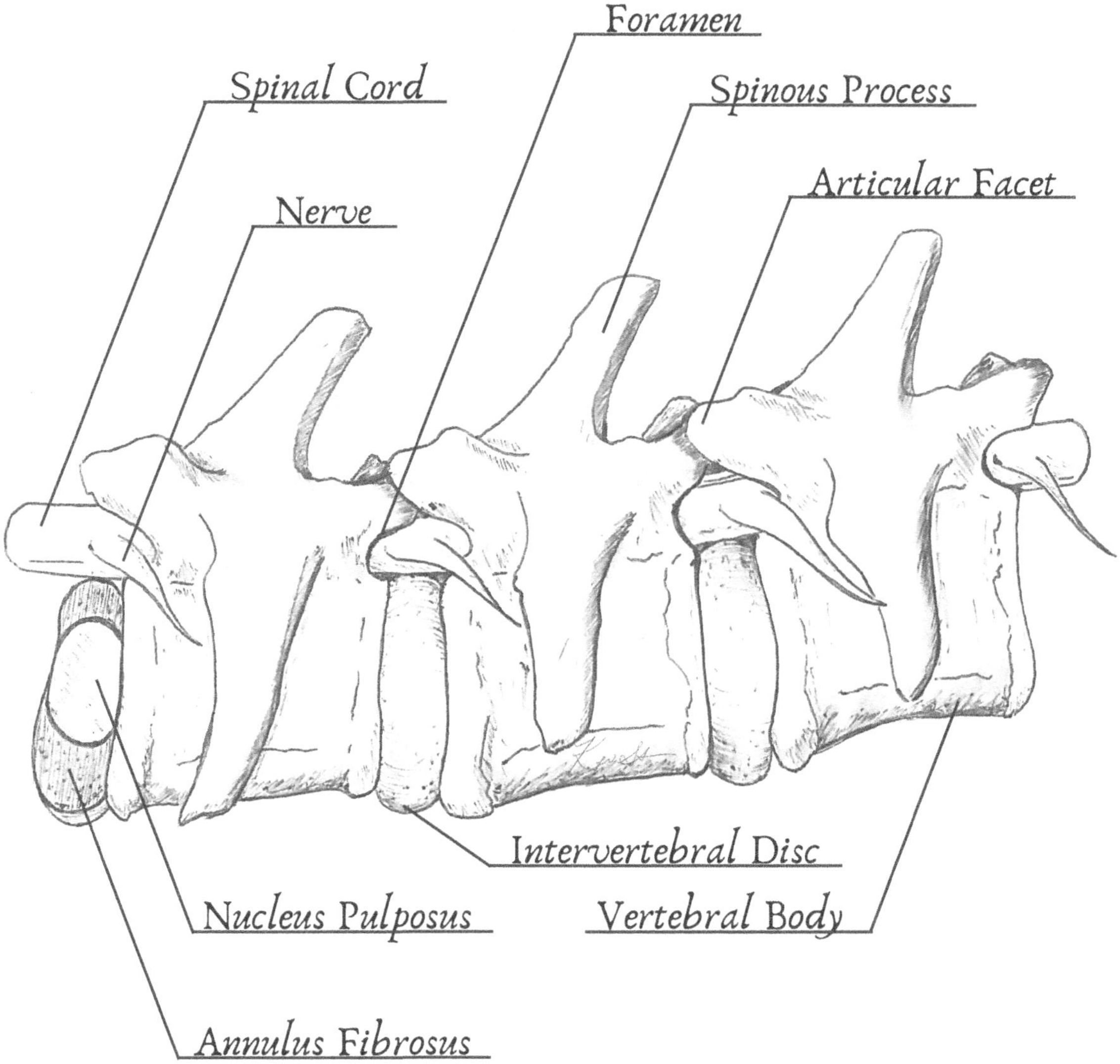

Vertebra: Lateral View

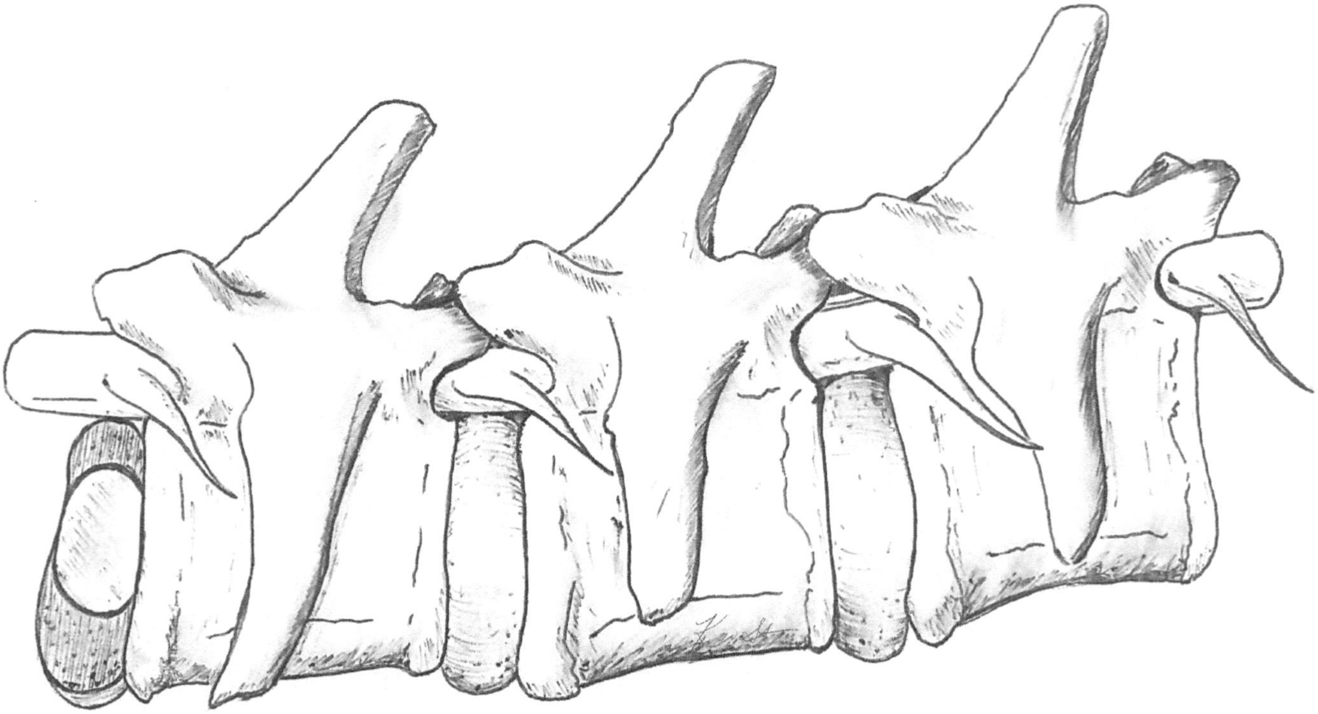

Lumbar Spine: Lateral View

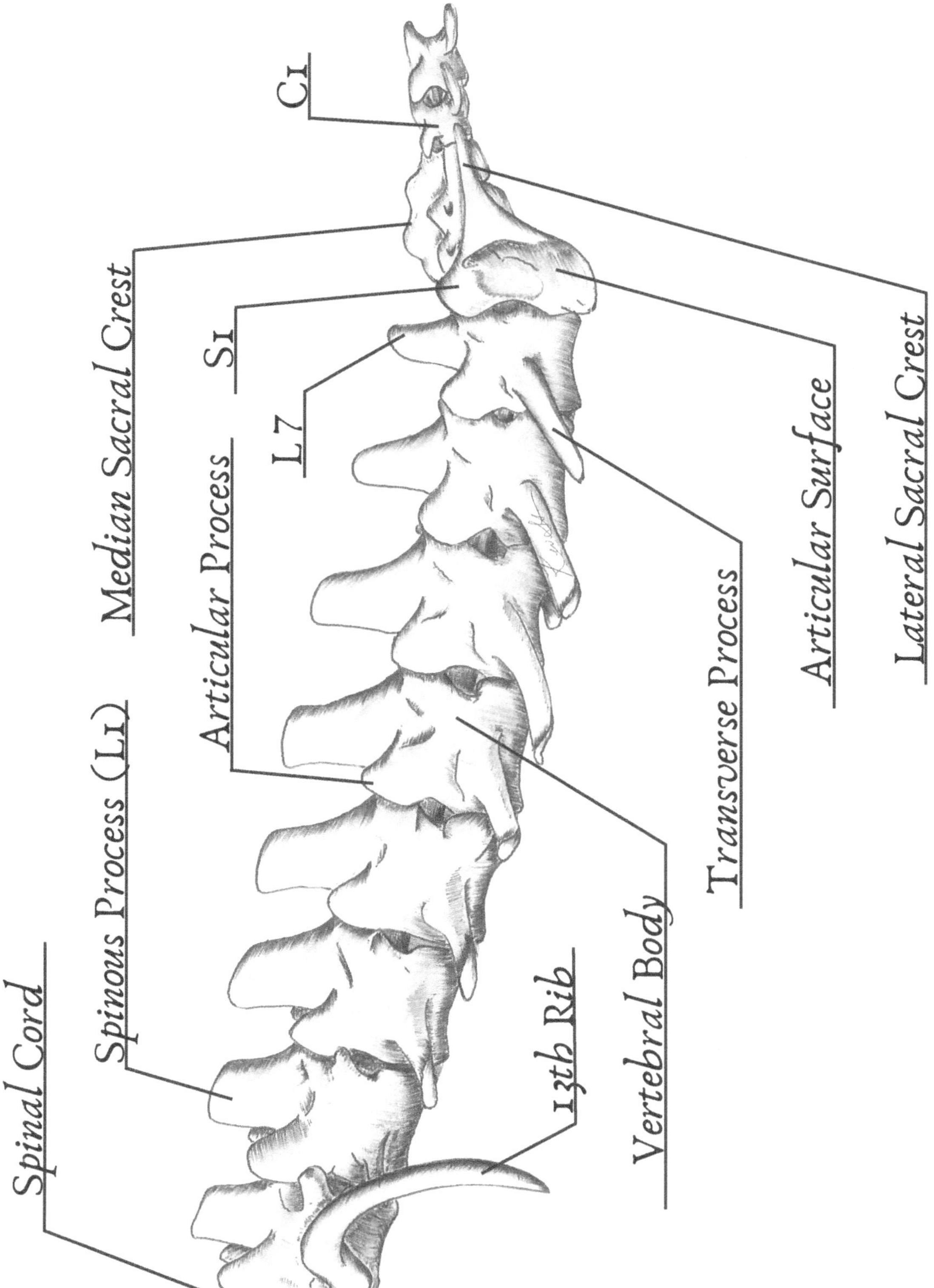

Lumbar Spine: Lateral View

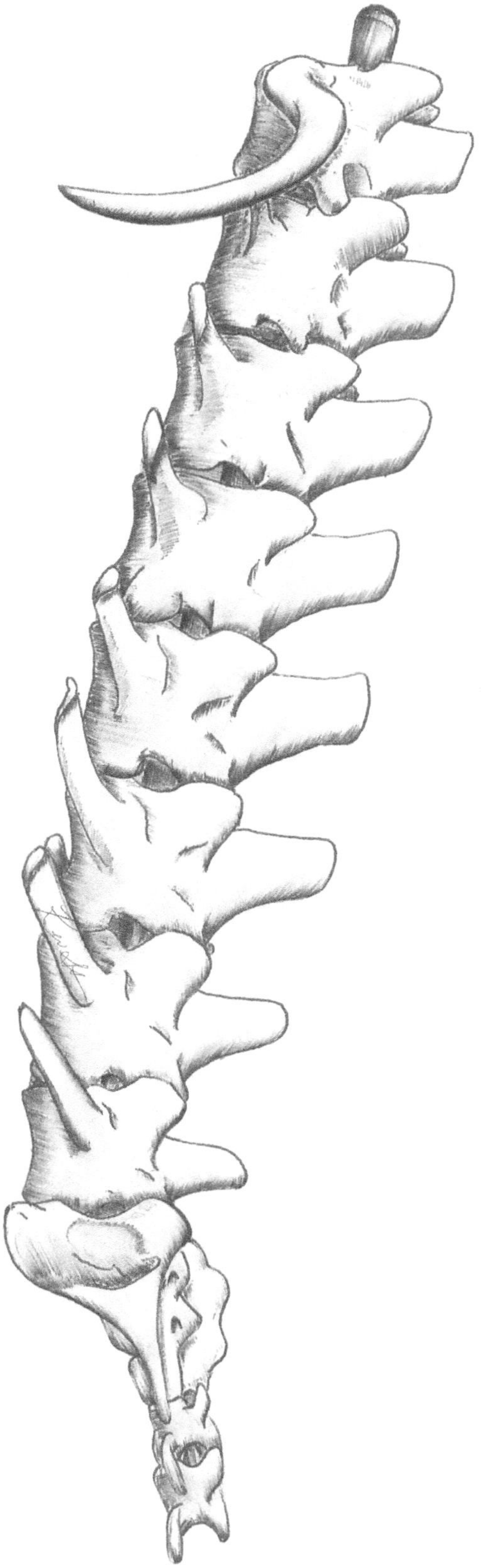

the Forelimb

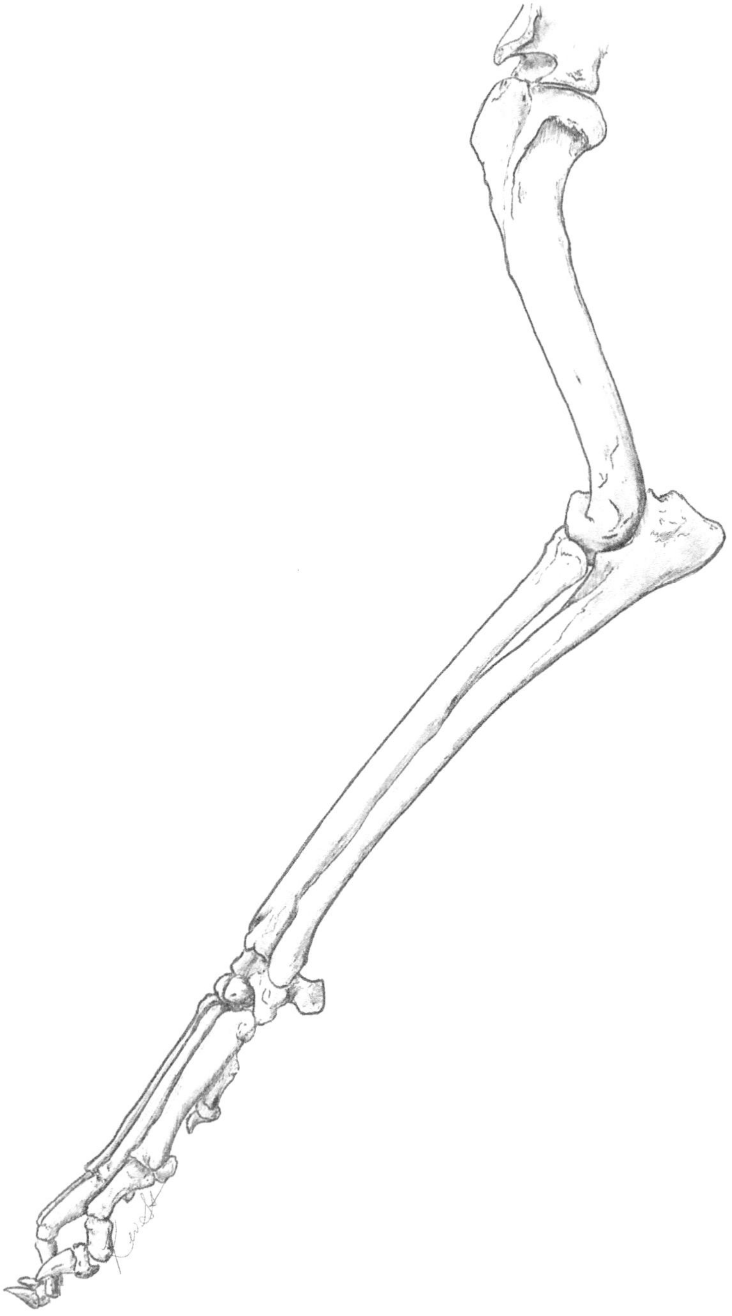

Notes:

- The forelimb is comprised of 29 bones.
- 25 of the forelimb bones are found in the carpus and foot.
- The shoulder joint is a ball and socket articulation between the humeral head and the glenoid cavity of the scapula.
- A dog's paw pads contain most of their sweat glands. Their only other sweat gland is in their nose.
- The elbow joint is a hinged articulation between the trochlea of the caudal humerus and the trochlear notch of the cranial ulna.
- A majority of canine forelimb injuries occur within the shoulder girdle.
- The arteries of the forelimb are the Axillary, Thoracodorsal, Brachial, Ulnar, Interosseous, Median, and Palmar arteries
- The veins of the forelimb are the Accessory Cephalic, Cephalic, Median, Median Cubital, Thoracodorsal, and Axillary vein.
- Elbow dysplasia describes an abnormal development of the joint due to medial compartment disease, osteochondritis dissecans, fragmented medial coronoid process, an ununited anconeal process, or a combination of these.

Shoulder: Lateral View

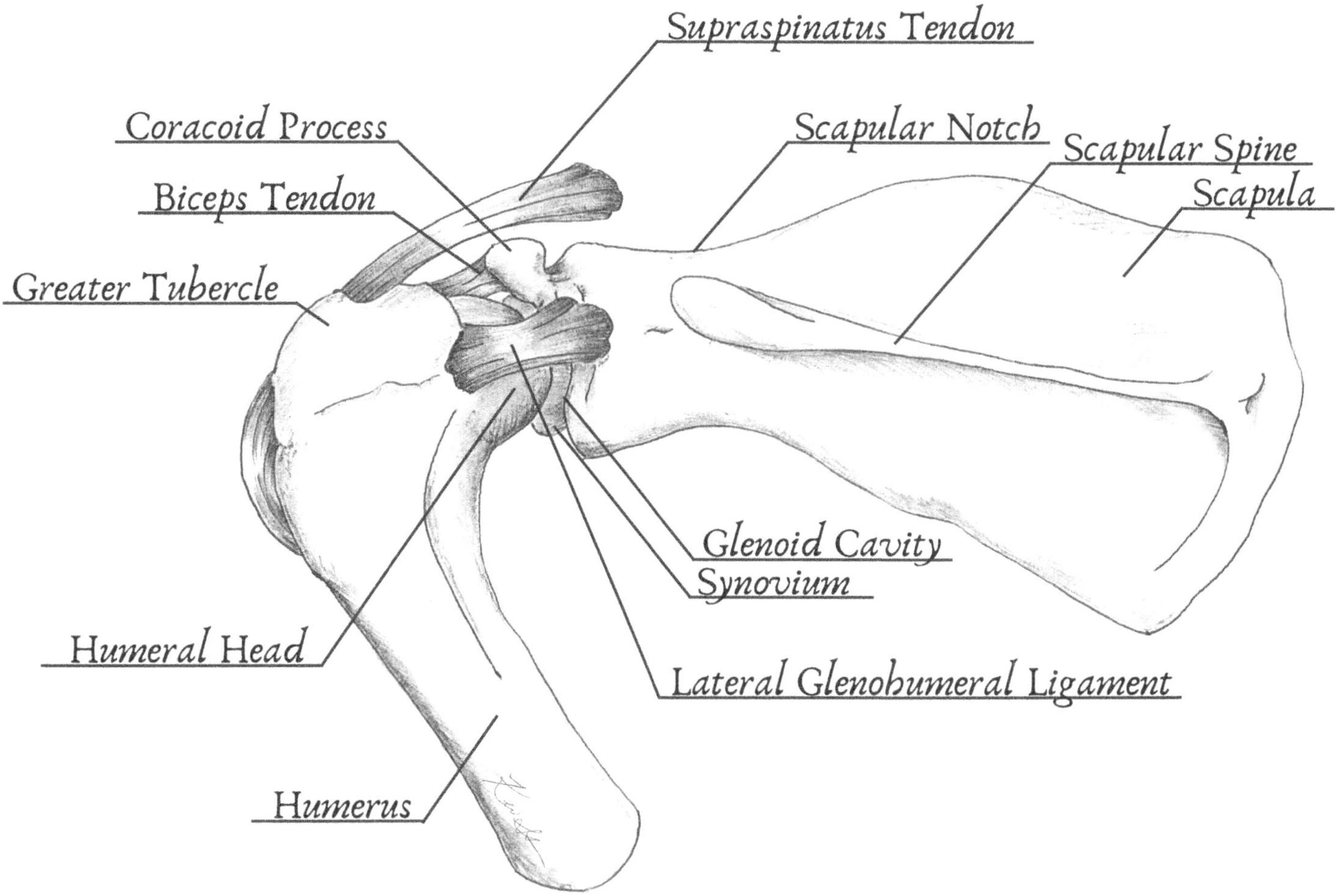

Shoulder: Lateral View

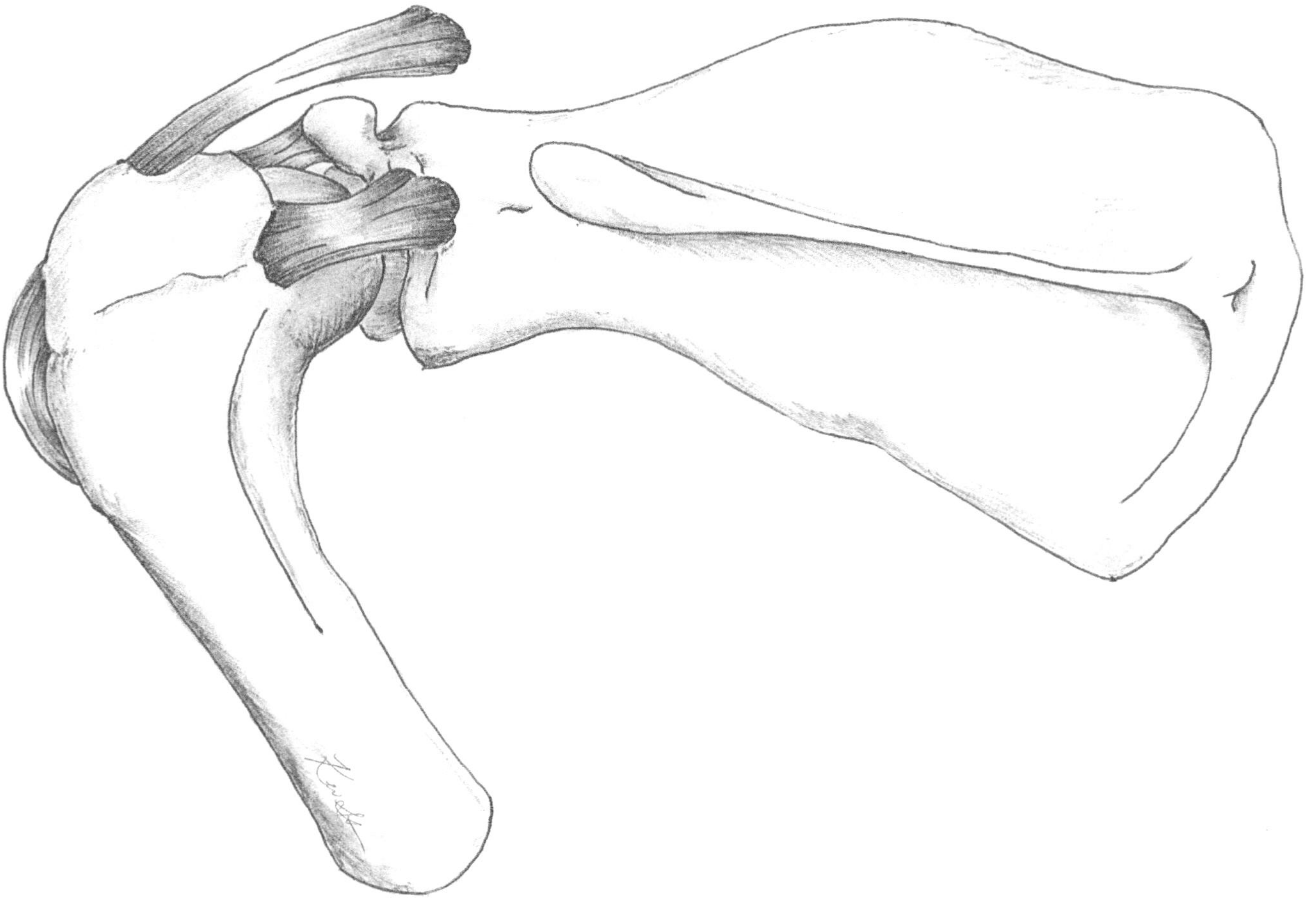

Humerus: Lateral View

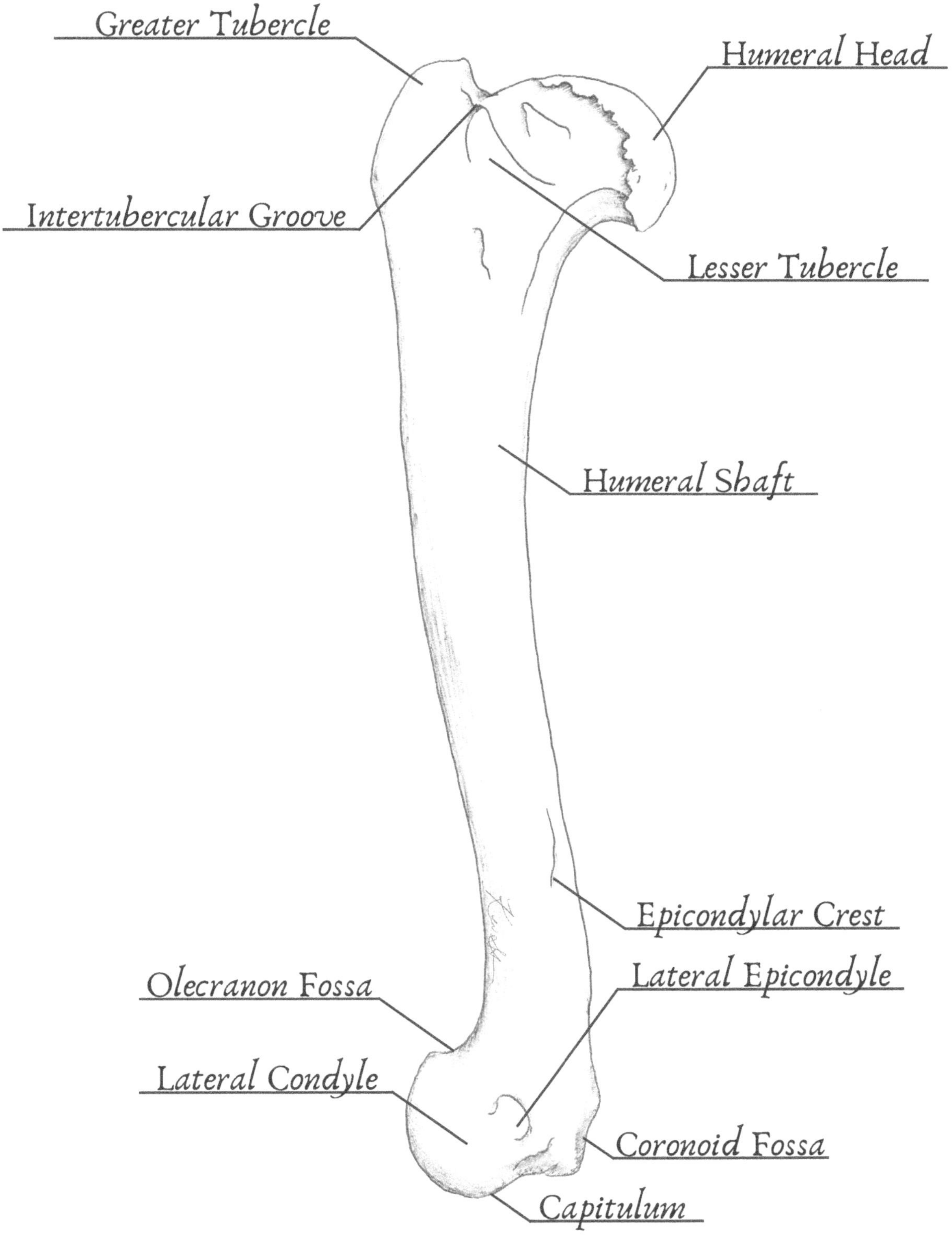

Humerus: Lateral View

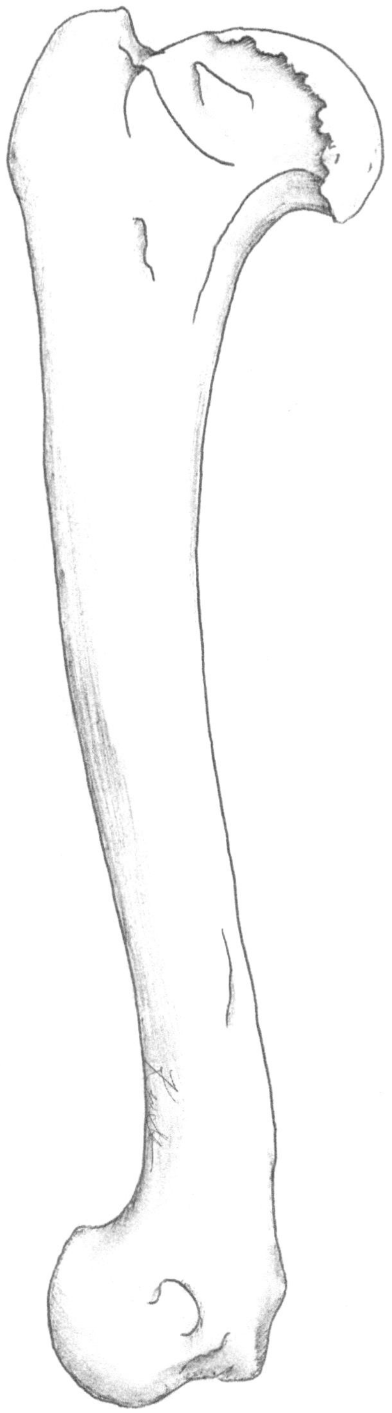

Humerus: Anterior View

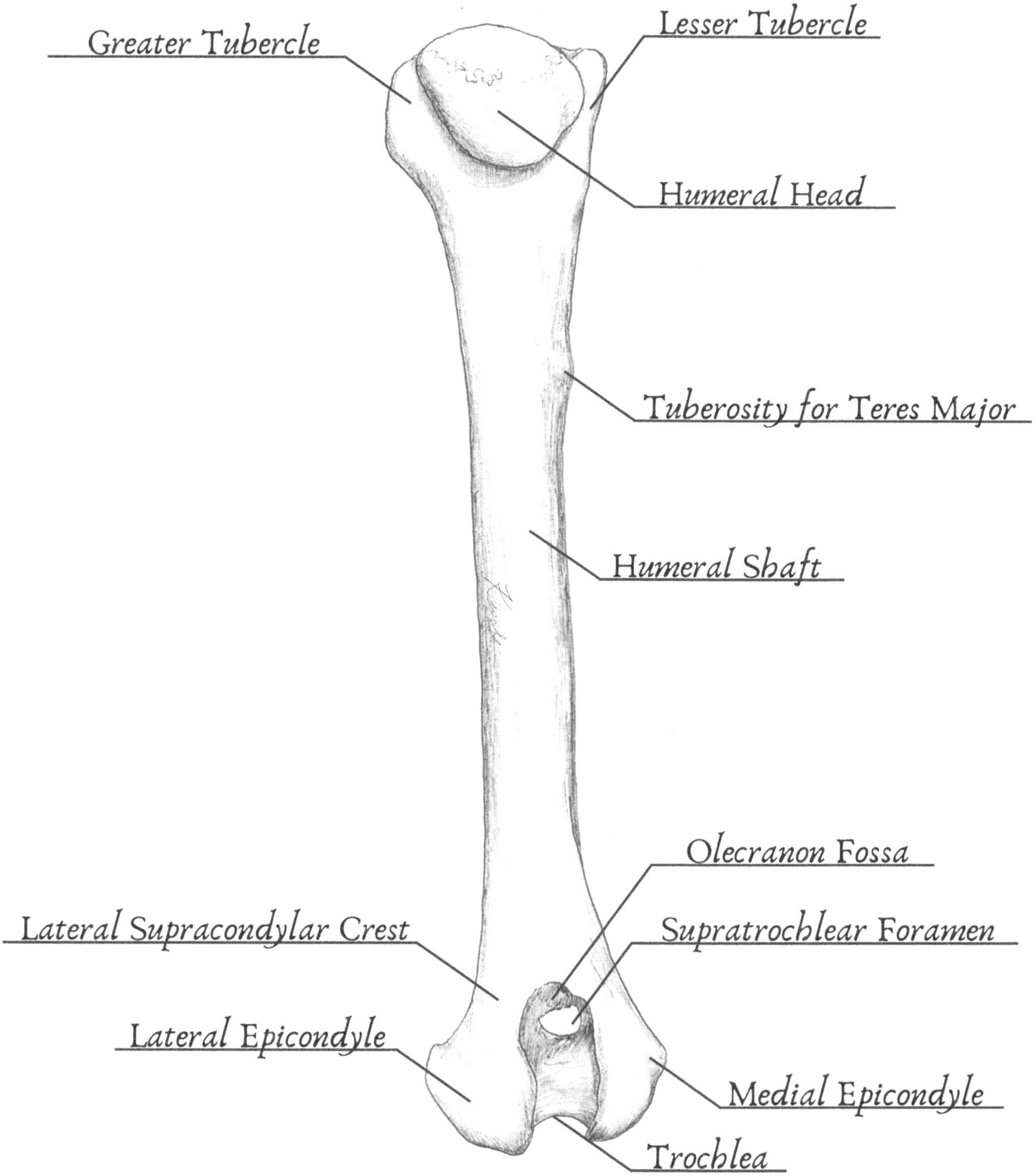

Humerus: Anterior View

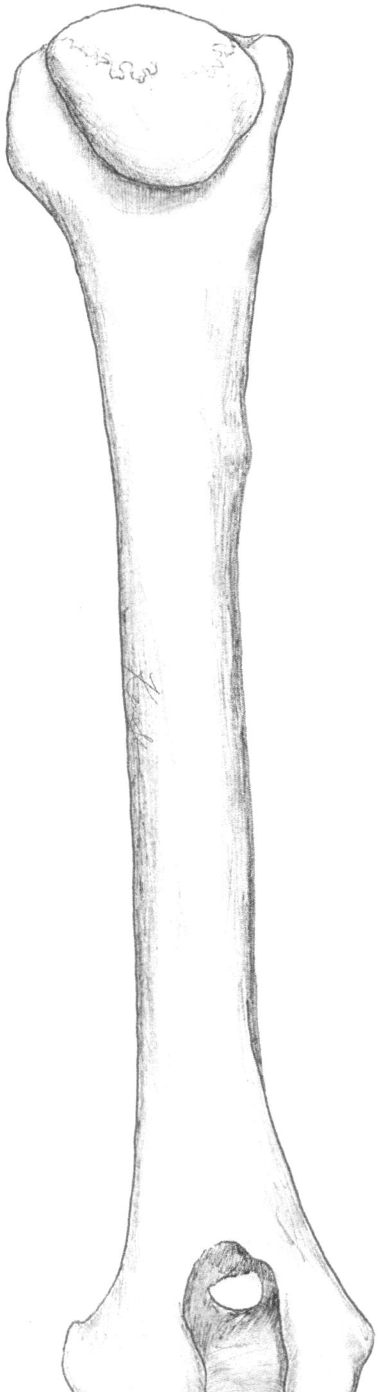

Elbow: Lateral View

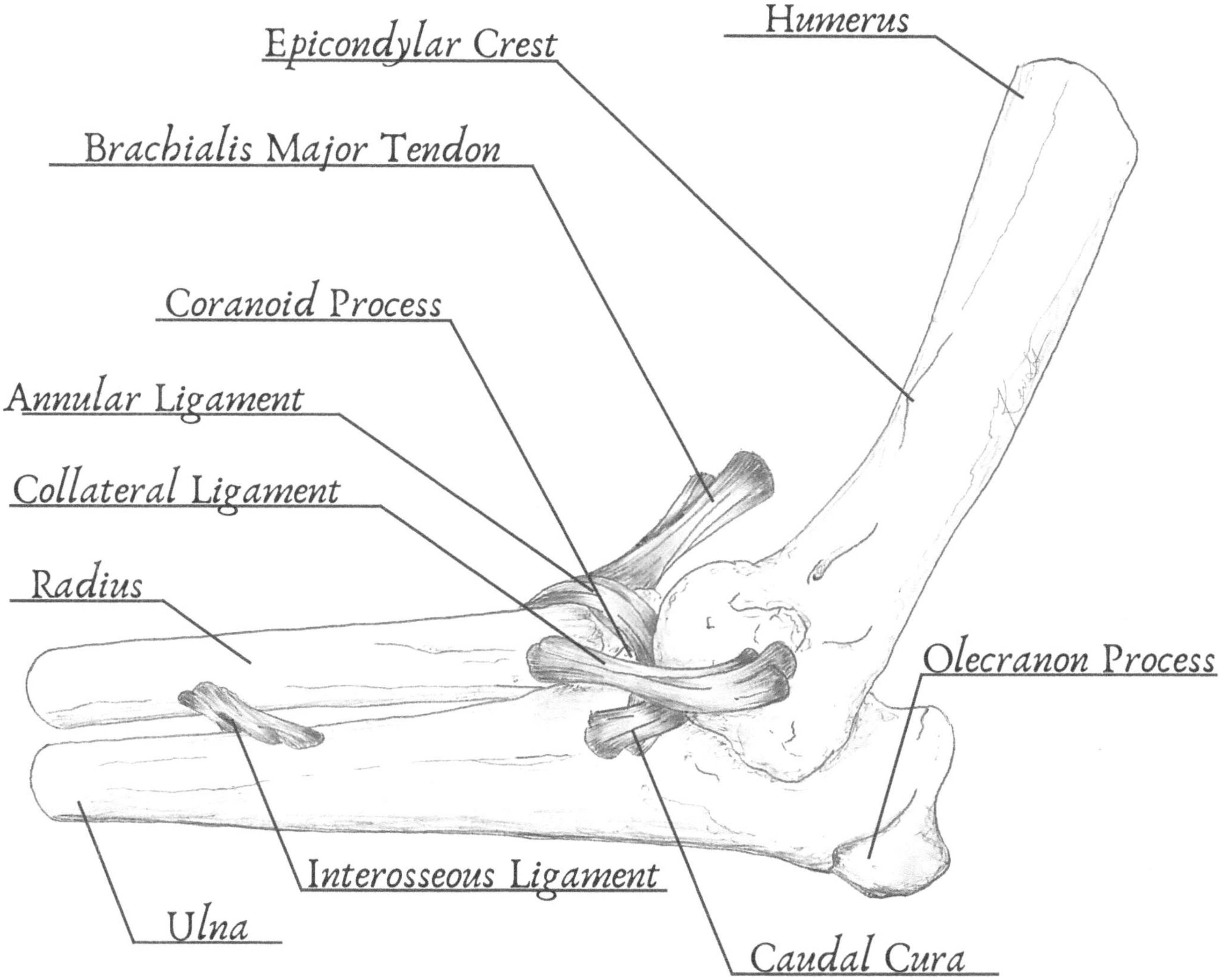

Elbow: Lateral View

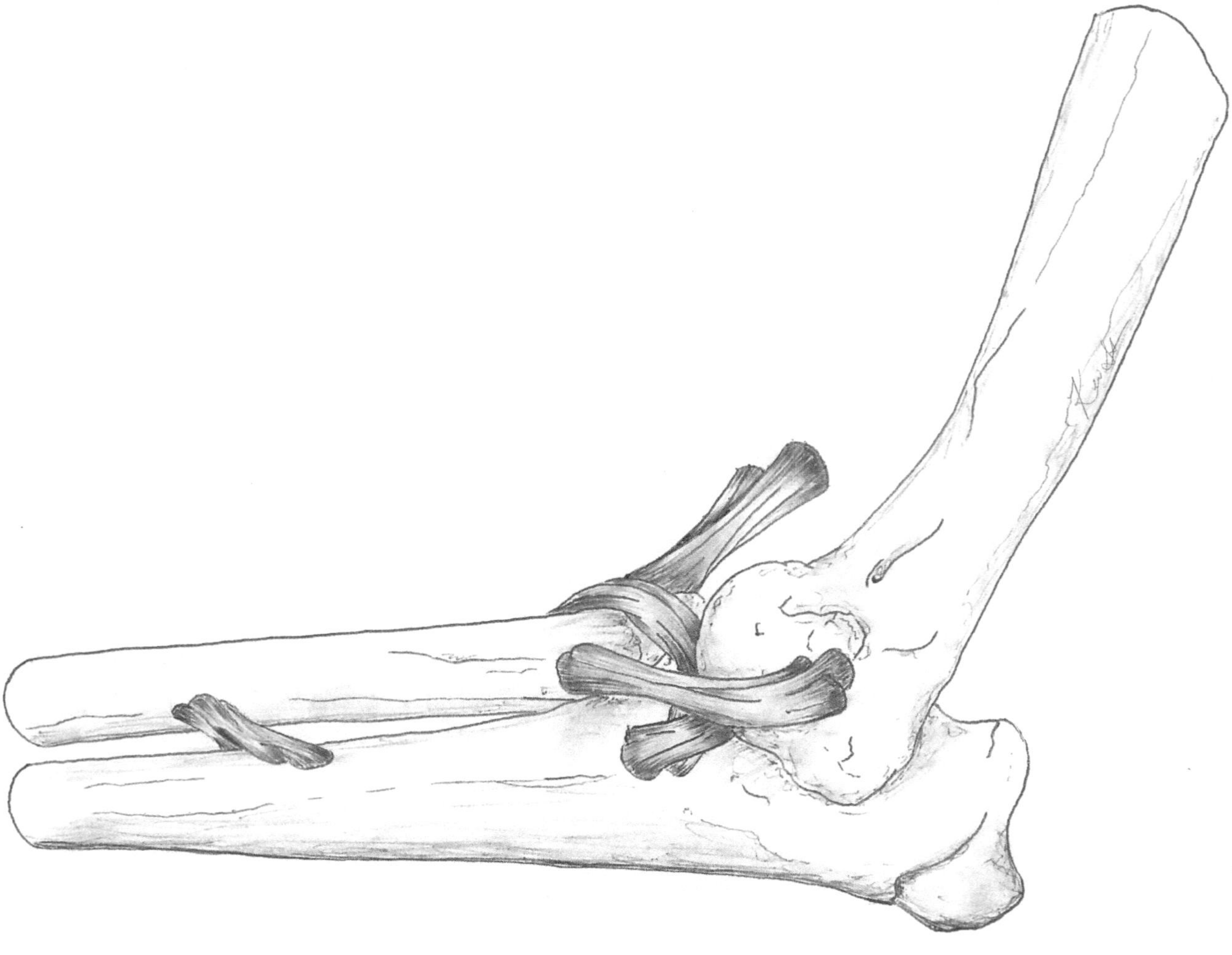

Radius & Ulna: Lateral View

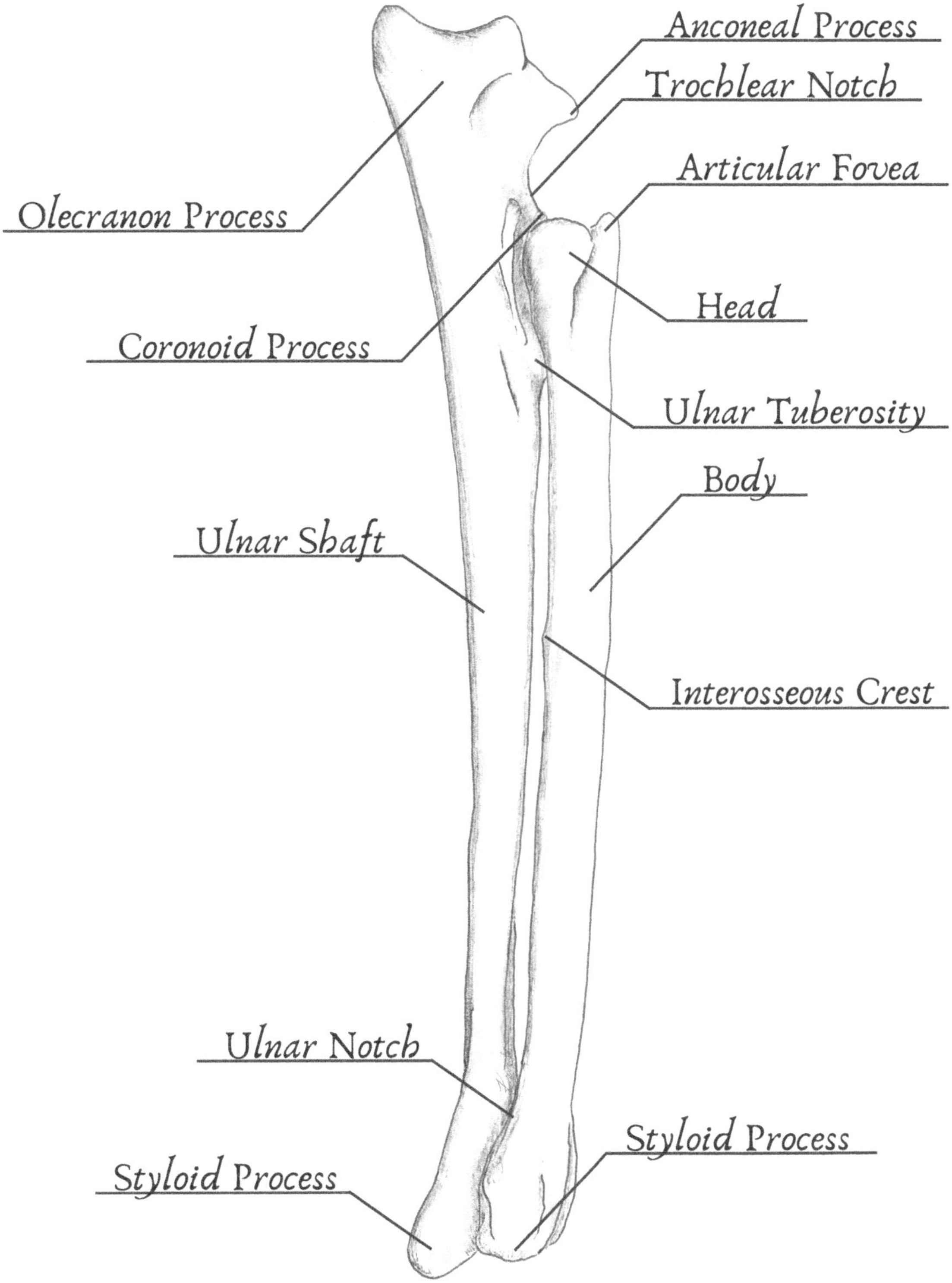

Radius & Ulna: Lateral View

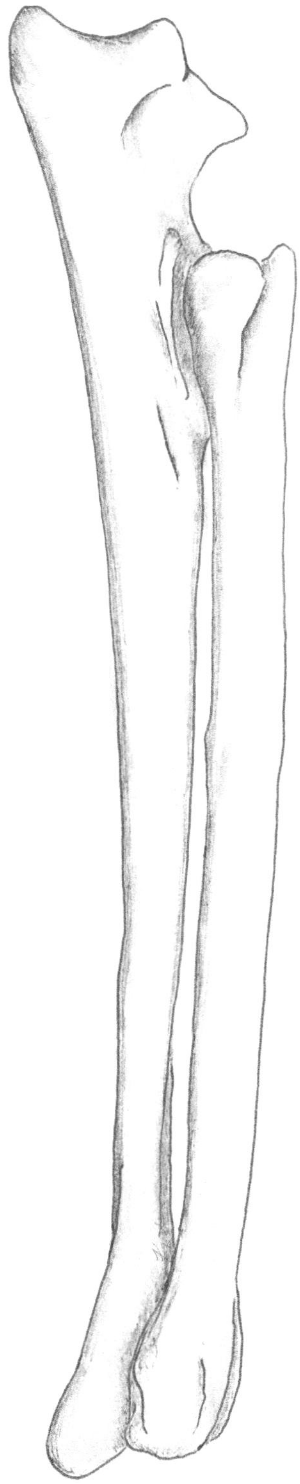

Carpus: Superior View

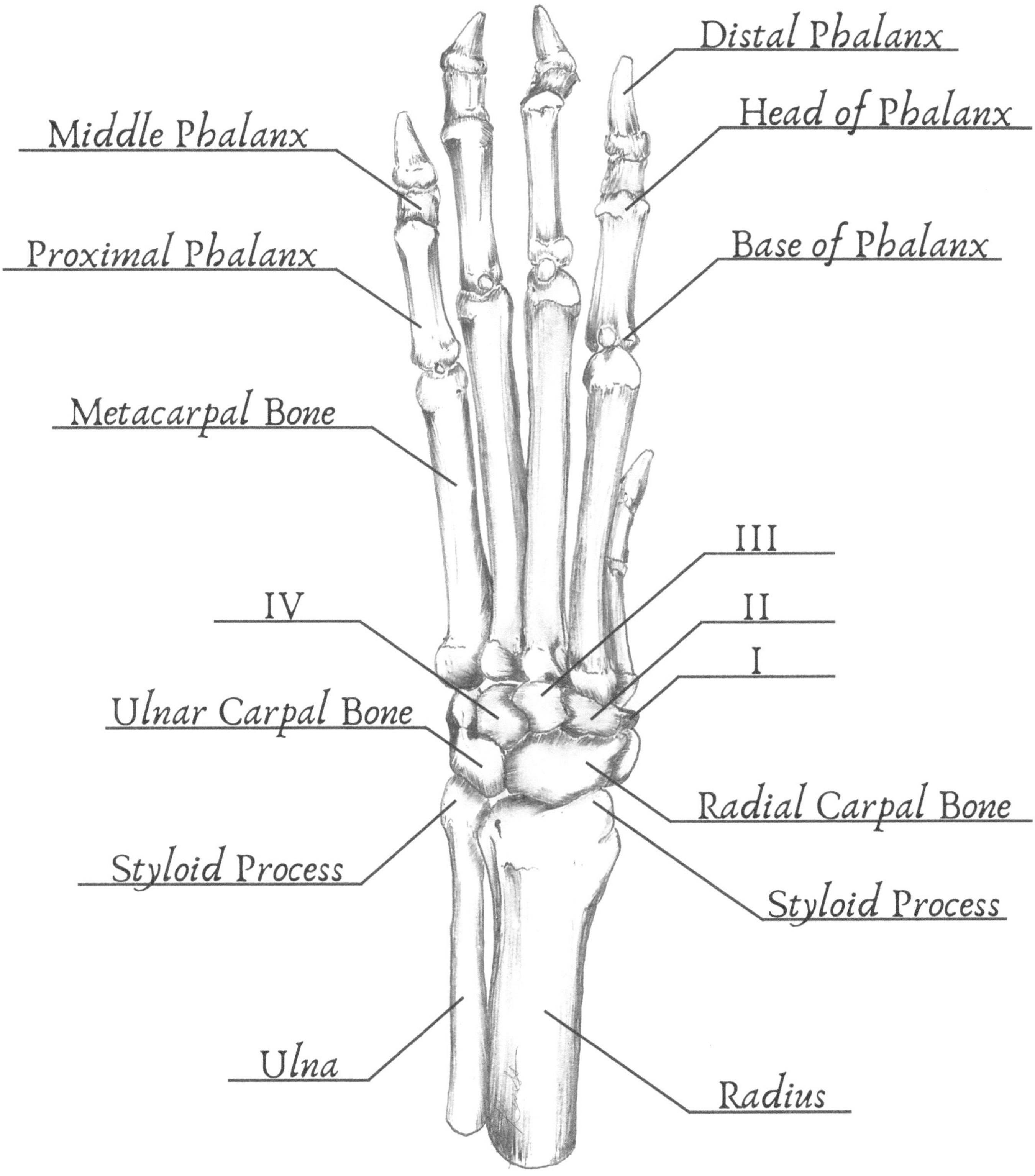

Carpus: Superior View

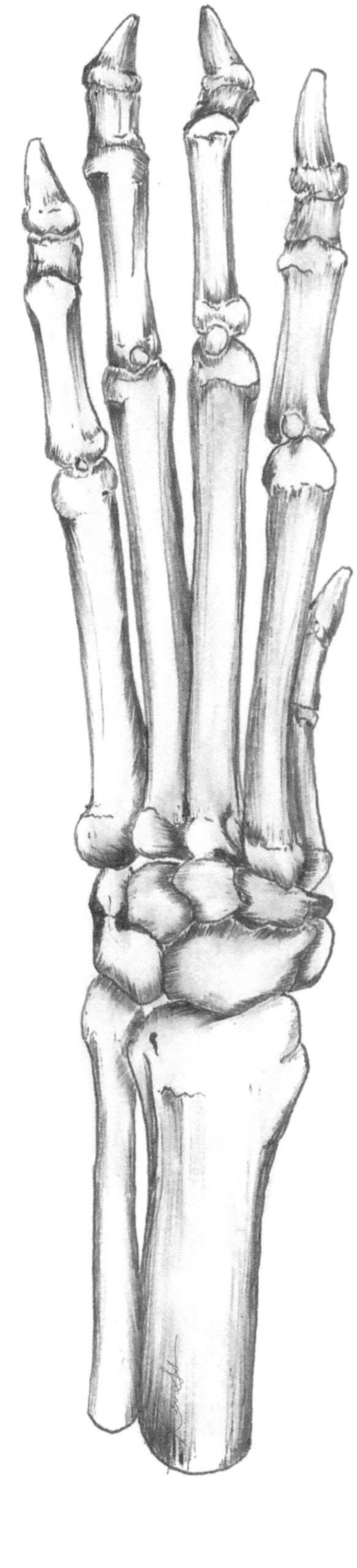

the Hindlimb

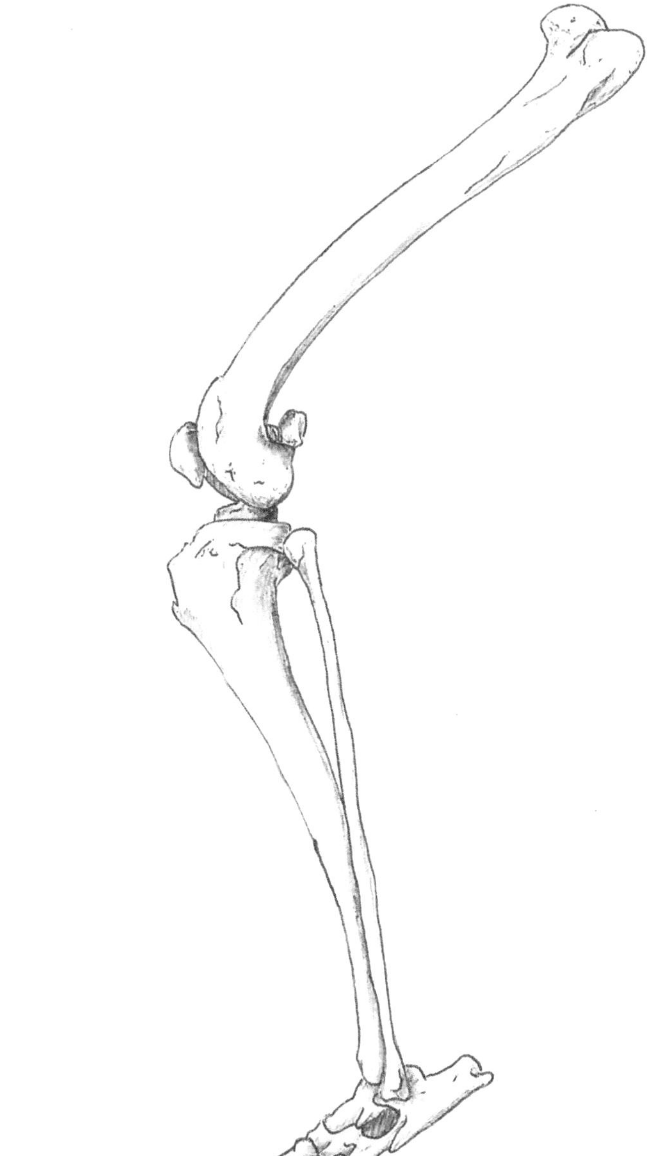

Notes:

- The hind limb is comprised of the pelvis, femur, patella, tibia, fibula, tarsals, metatarsals, and phalanges.
- The hip joint is a ball and socket articulation between the femoral head and the acetabulum of the pelvis.
- The stifle joint is a hinged articulation between the femur and the tibia.
- The primary arteries of the hindlimb are the aorta, external and internal iliac, deep femoral, femoral, saphenous, popliteal, cranial tibial, dorsal pedal, and perforating ramus.
- The primary veins of the hindlimb are the lateral saphenous and caudal branches, medial saphenous and caudal branches, cranial tibial, popliteal, femoral, external and internal iliac, caudal vena cava.
- Between articular surfaces of the femur and tibia is a cartilage structure known as the meniscus.
- The sacro-iliac (SI) joint, is the articulation between the sacral spine and the ilium of the pelvis.
- The Caudal and Cranial cruciate ligaments are a common site for injury among canines.
- A dog may have up to 44 sesamoid bones in their body. Sesamoids are ossifications embedded in the tendons, the largest of which is the patella.

Pelvis: Anterior View

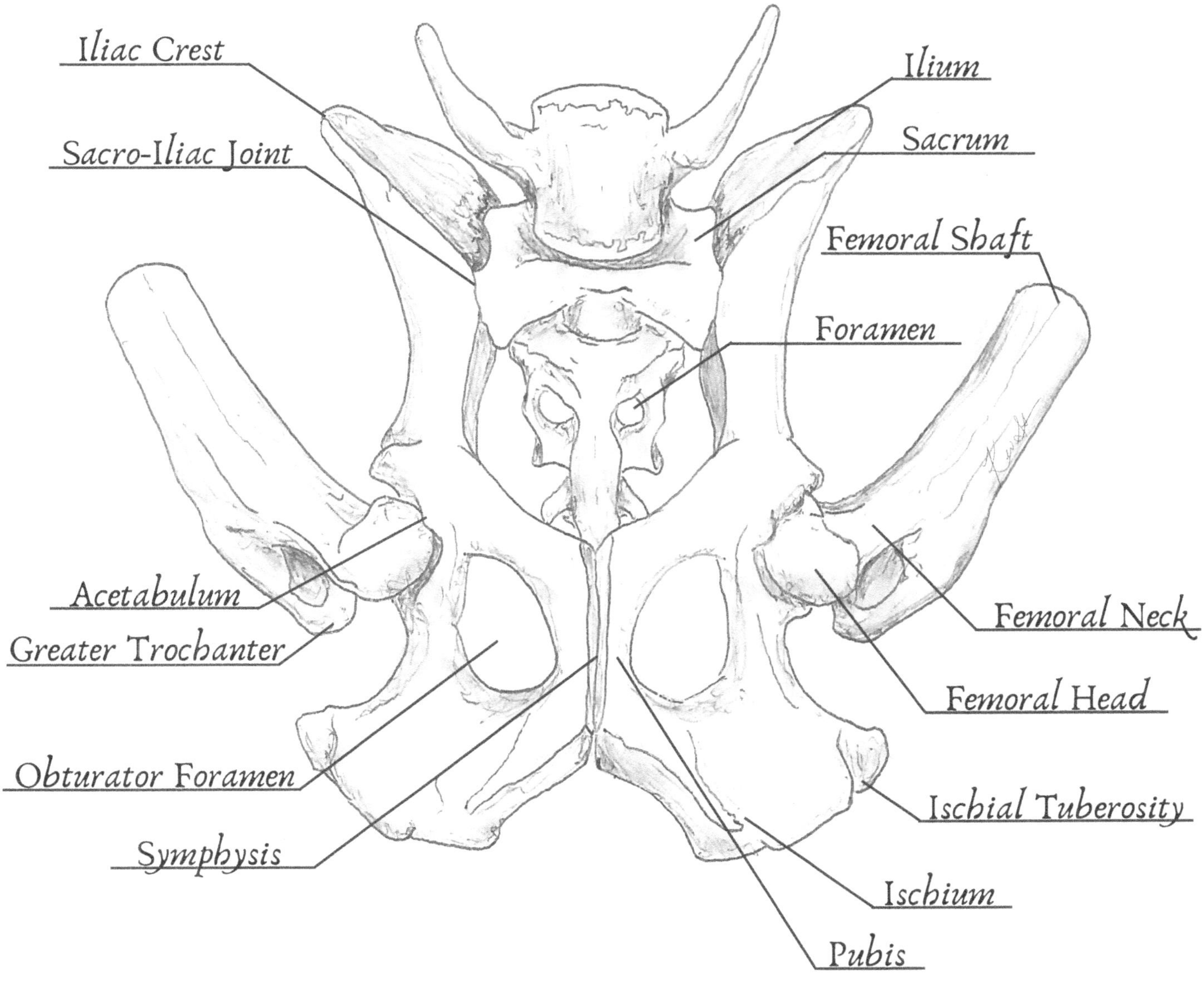

Pelvis: Anterior View

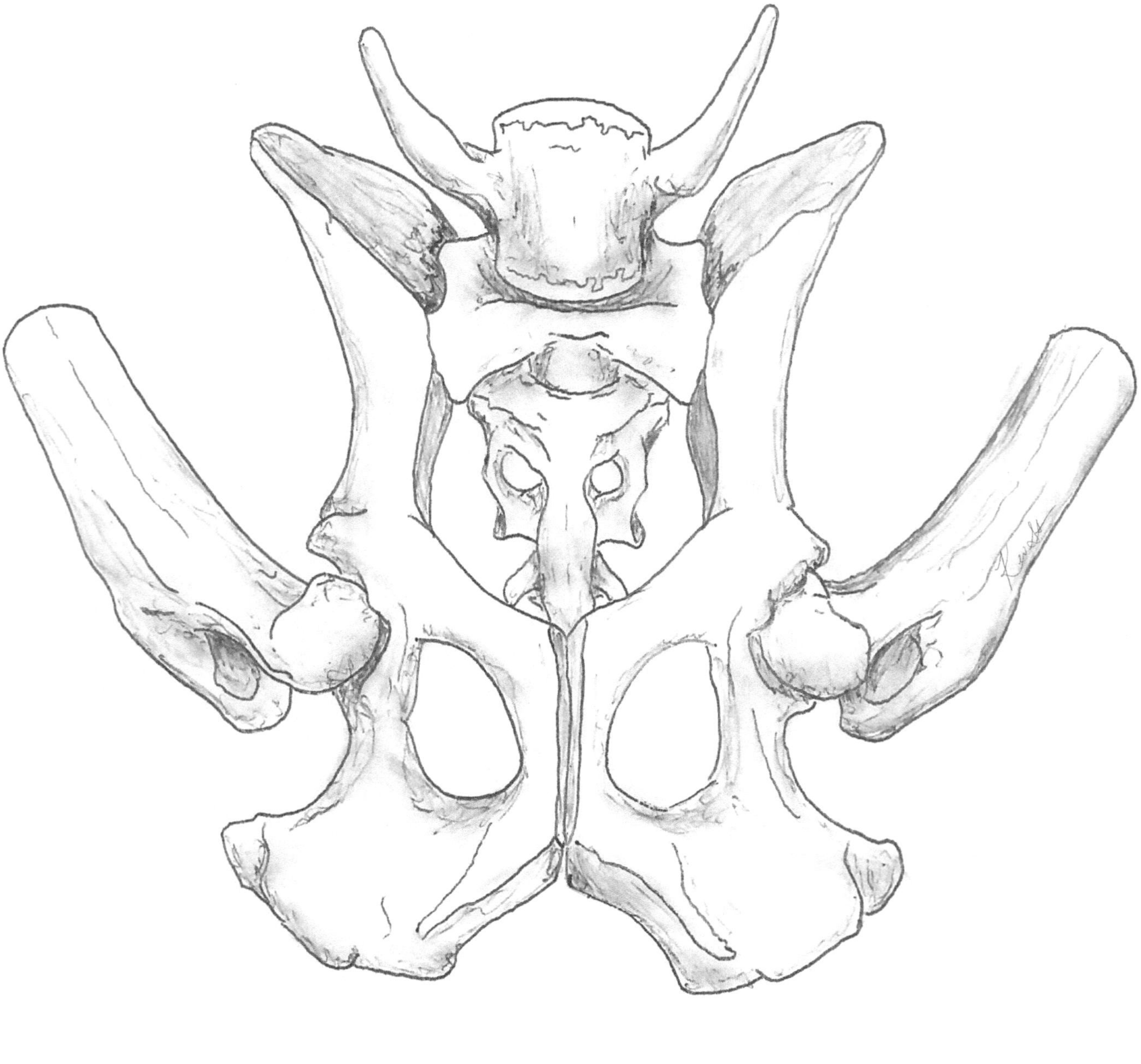

Femur: Anterior View

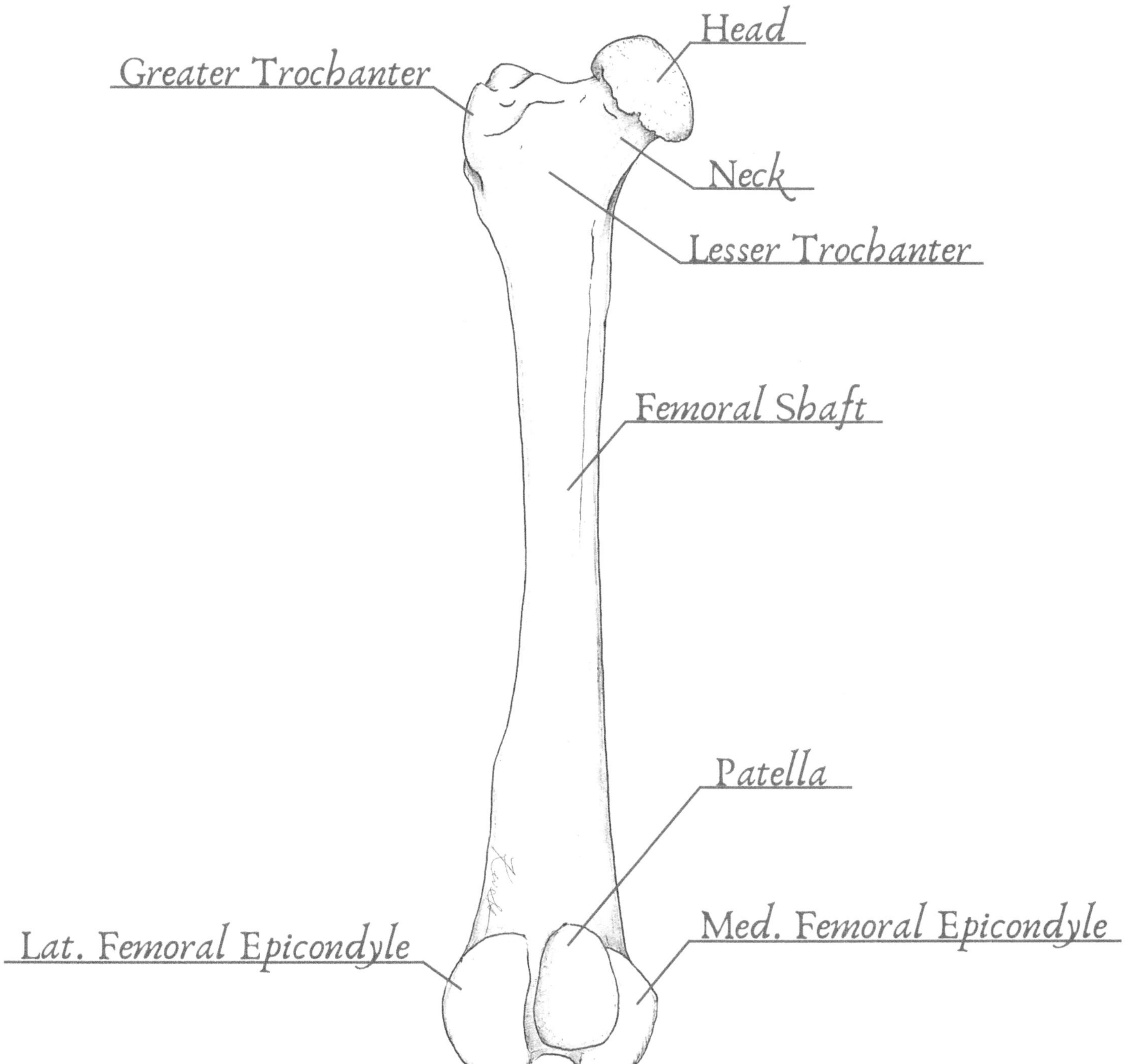

Femur: Anterior View

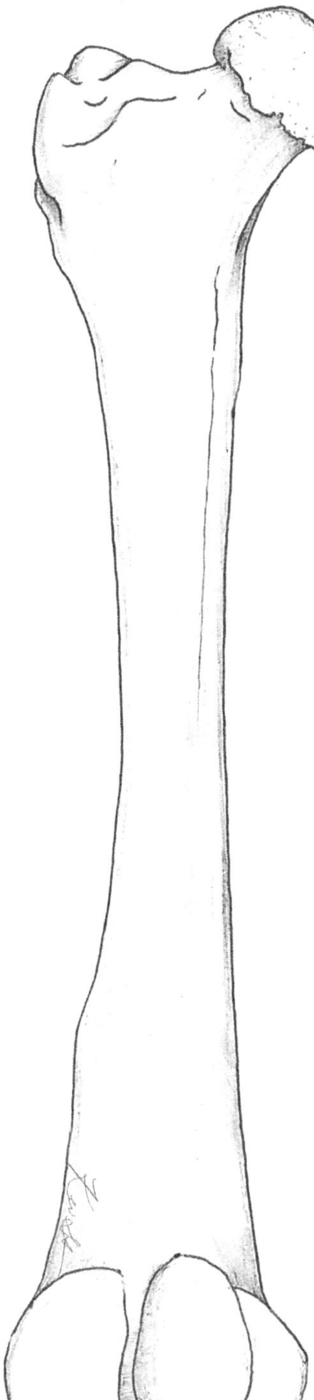

Stifle: Lateral View

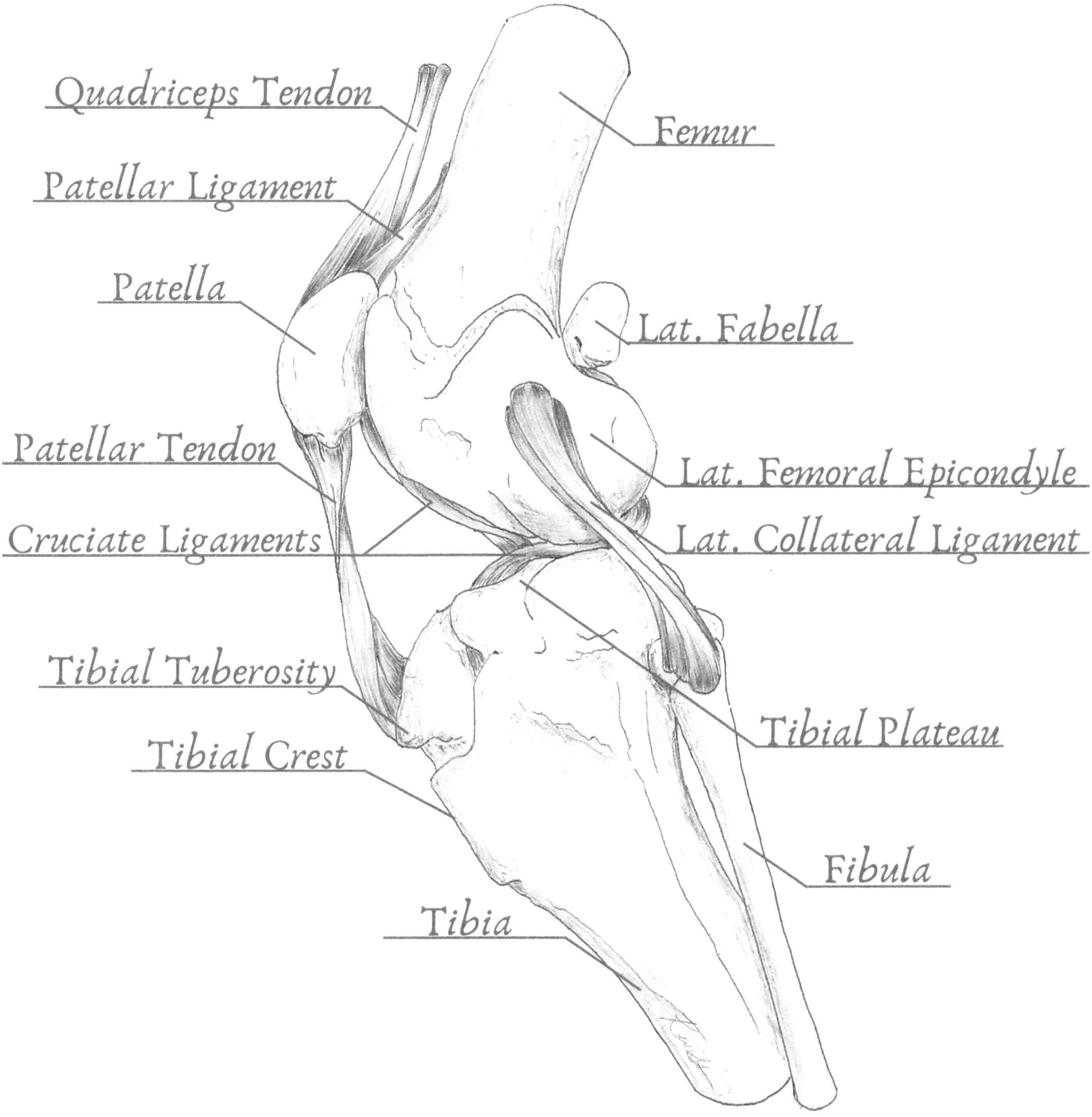

Stifle: Lateral View

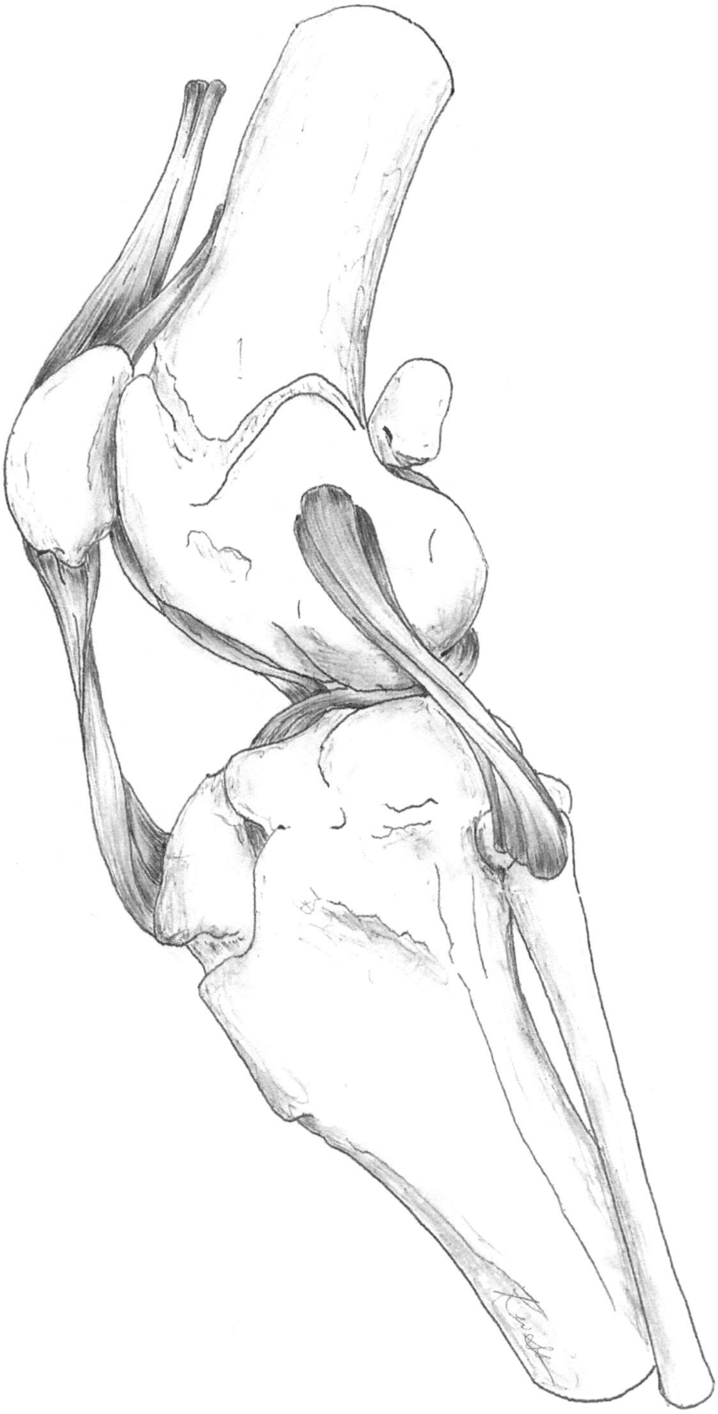

Stifle: Anterior View

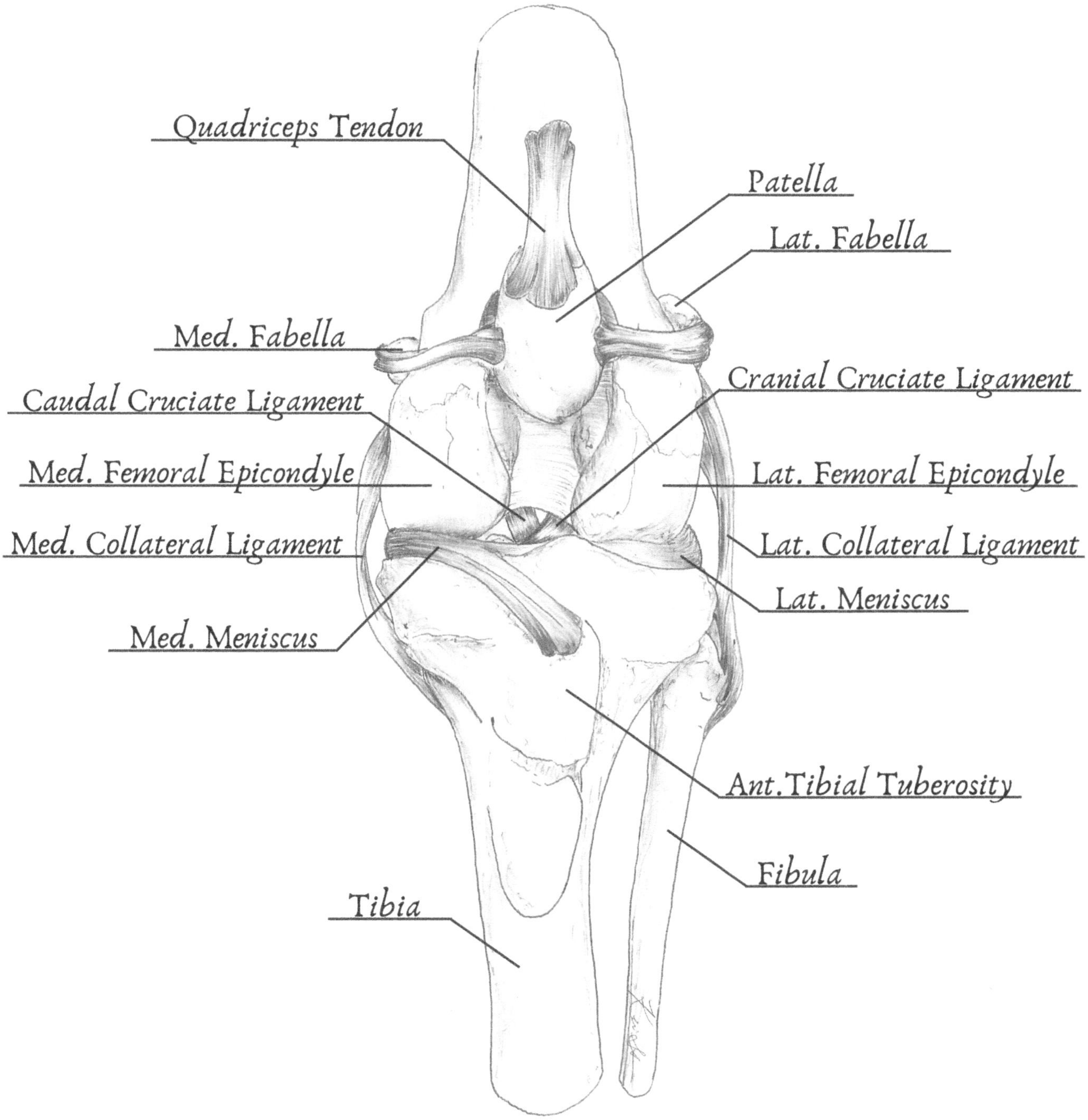

Stifle: Anterior View

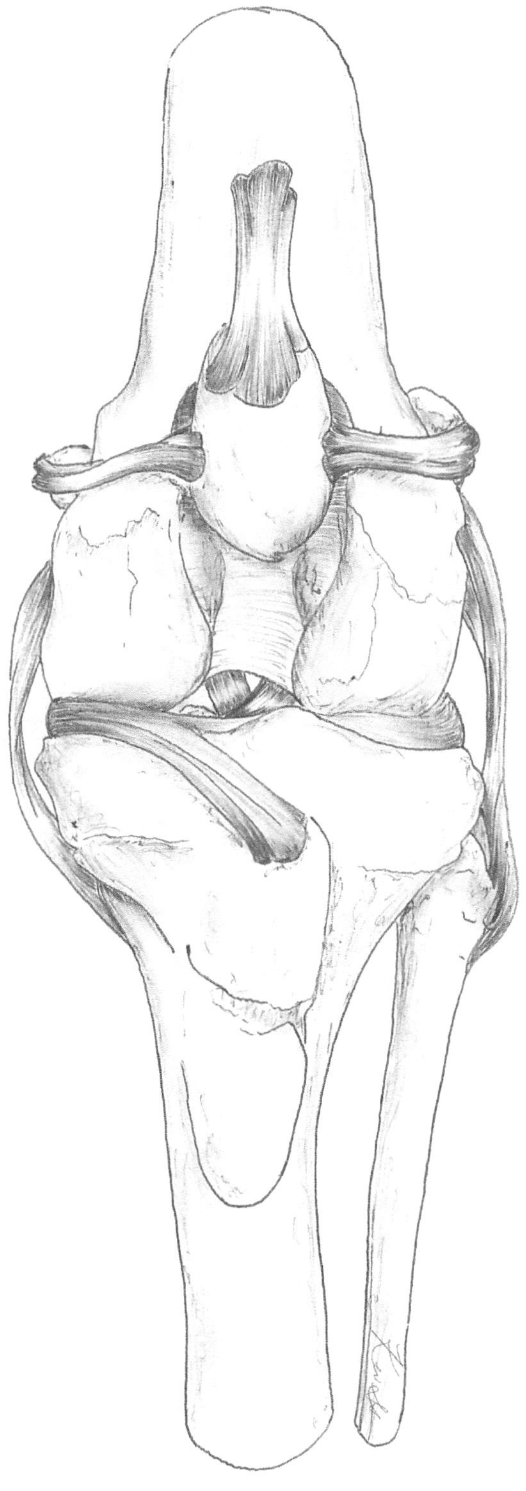

Tibia & Fibula: Anterior View

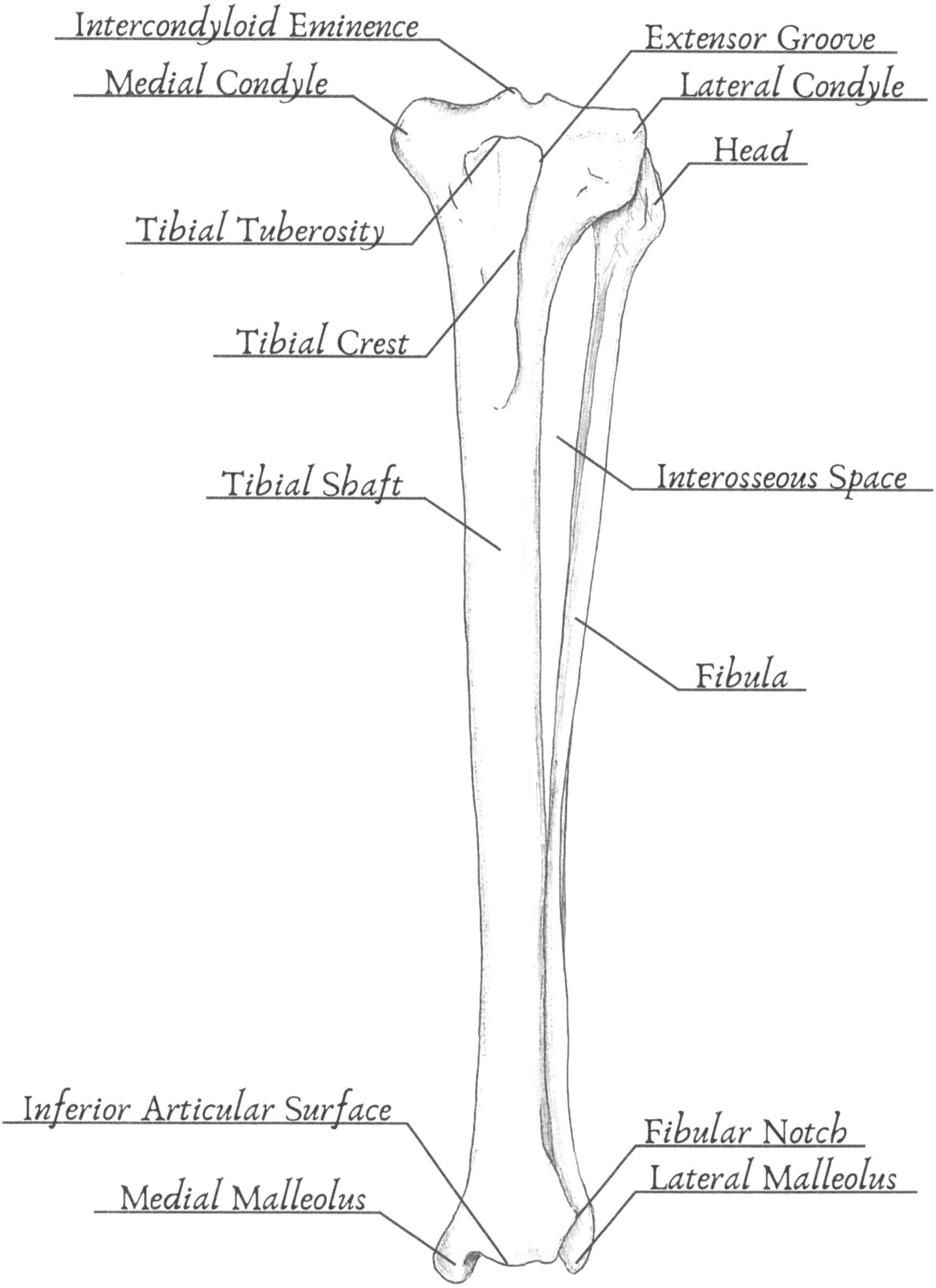

Tibia & Fibula: Anterior View

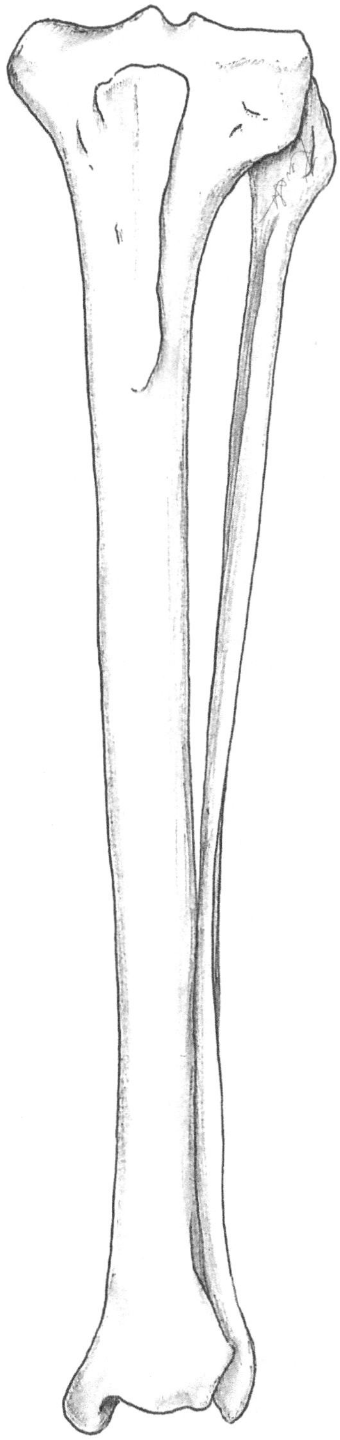

Tarsus: Lateral View

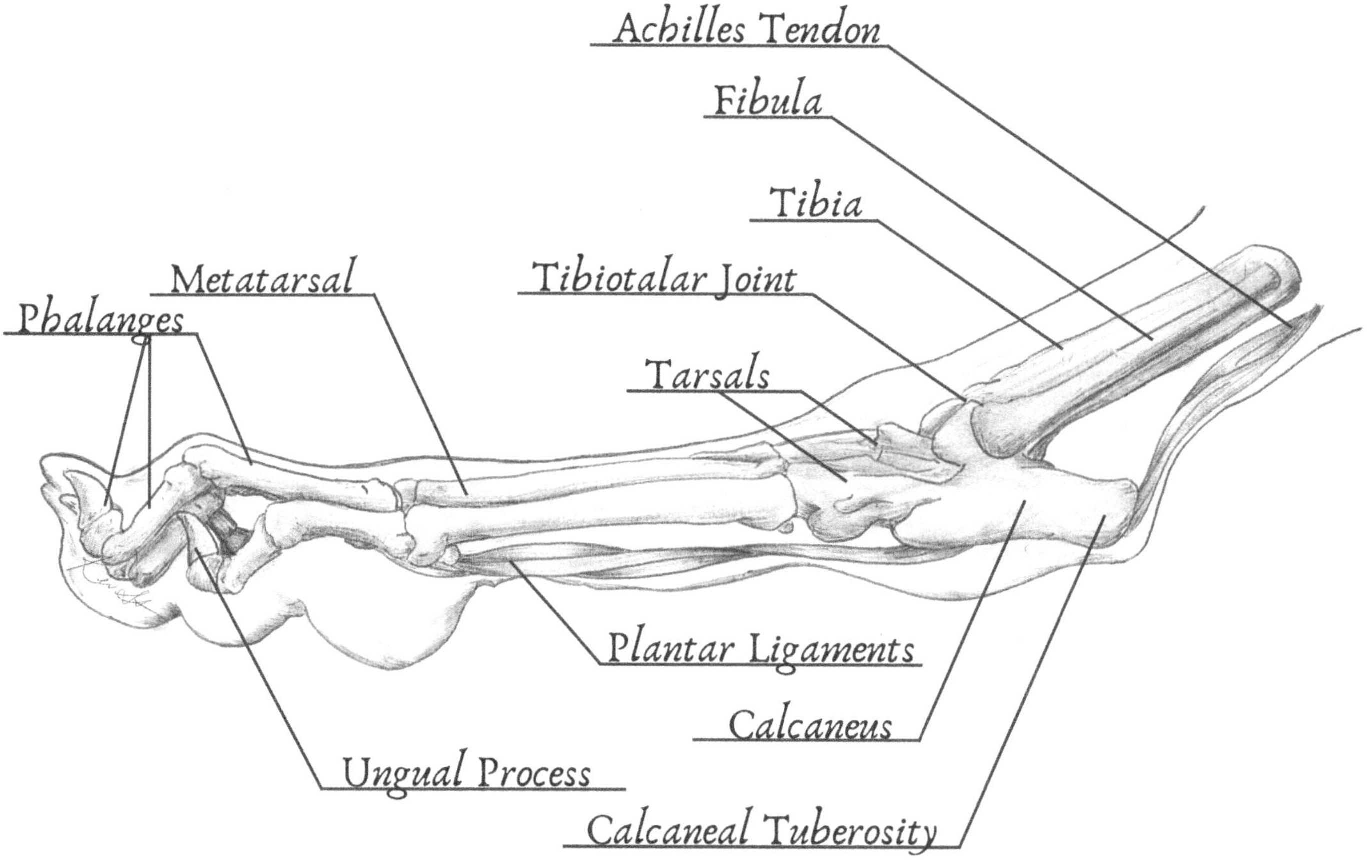

Tarsus: Lateral View

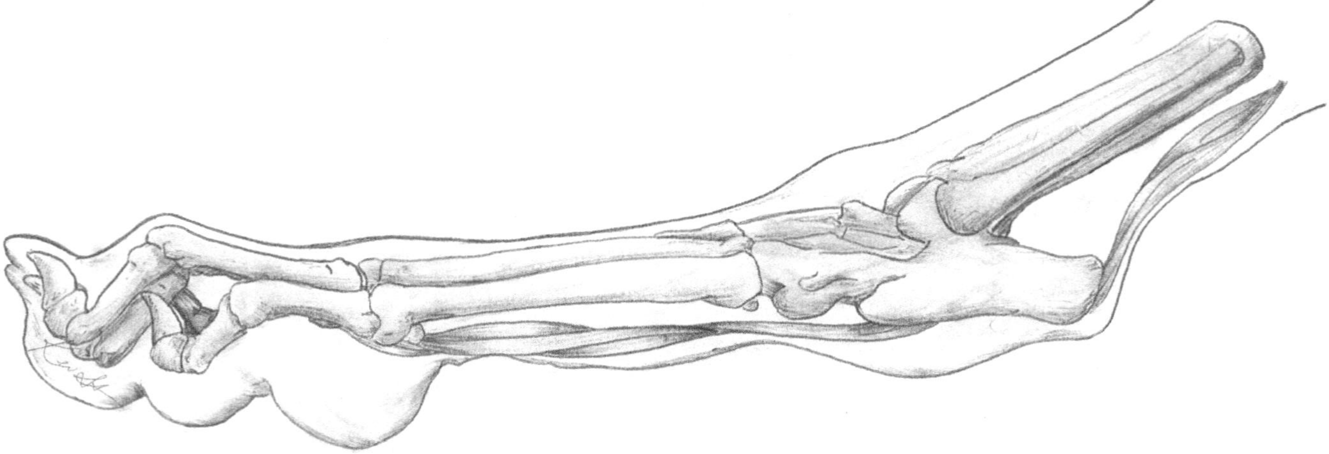

the Thorax

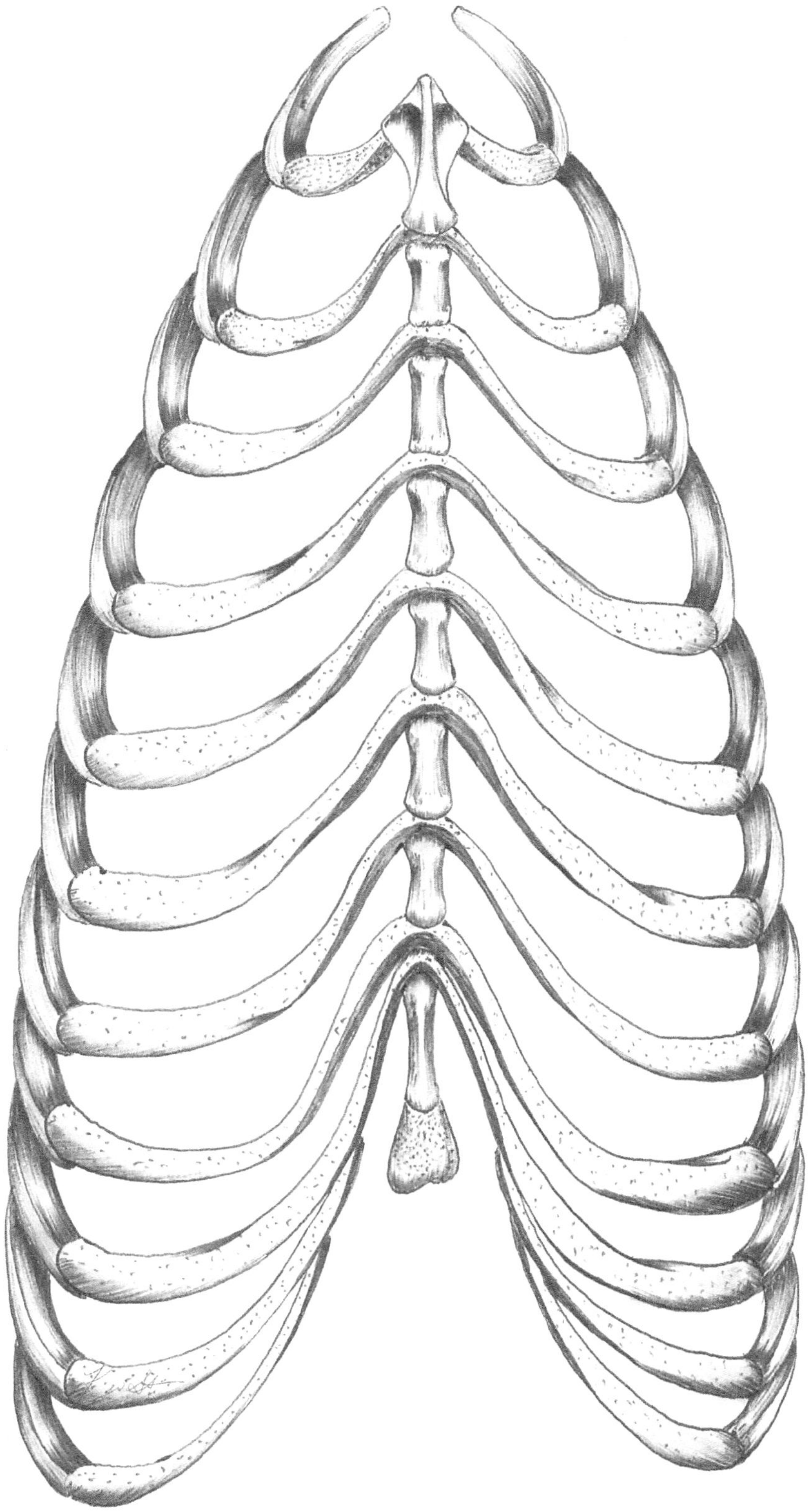

Notes:

- There are 2 separate lobes in the left lung and 3 separate lobes in the right.
- The airway path: oropharynx, larynx, trachea, Main stem bronchus, secondary bronchus, tertiary bronchus, bronchioles, alveoli (air sacs).
- The alveolar air sacs transport gasses between the lungs and blood vessels.
- Between the lungs and the chest wall is a protective layer called the pleura. It consists of two membranes (the parietal pleura and the visceral pleura) with a space between called the pleural cavity.
- Cardiopulmonary circulatory path: Inferior or Superior Vena Cava, Right Atrium, Tricuspid Valve, Right Ventricle, Pulmonary Valve, Pulmonary Arteries, Pulmonary Veins, Left Atrium, Mitral Valve, Left Ventricle, Aortic Valve, Aorta
- A normal heart rate for a dog can be between 70-120 BPM depending on the breed, size, and age of the dog.
- The thorax contains 13 pairs of ribs. The last two pairs are called "floating ribs" as they do not connect ventrally to a costal cartilage.
- Electrical impulses to the heart are created and controlled by the Sinoatrial (SA) Node, Atrioventricular (AV) Node, and the Bundle of His.
- The thorax also contains a collar bone, however it is a floating bone and does not connect to the shoulder or sternum.

Ribs & Sternum: Anterior View

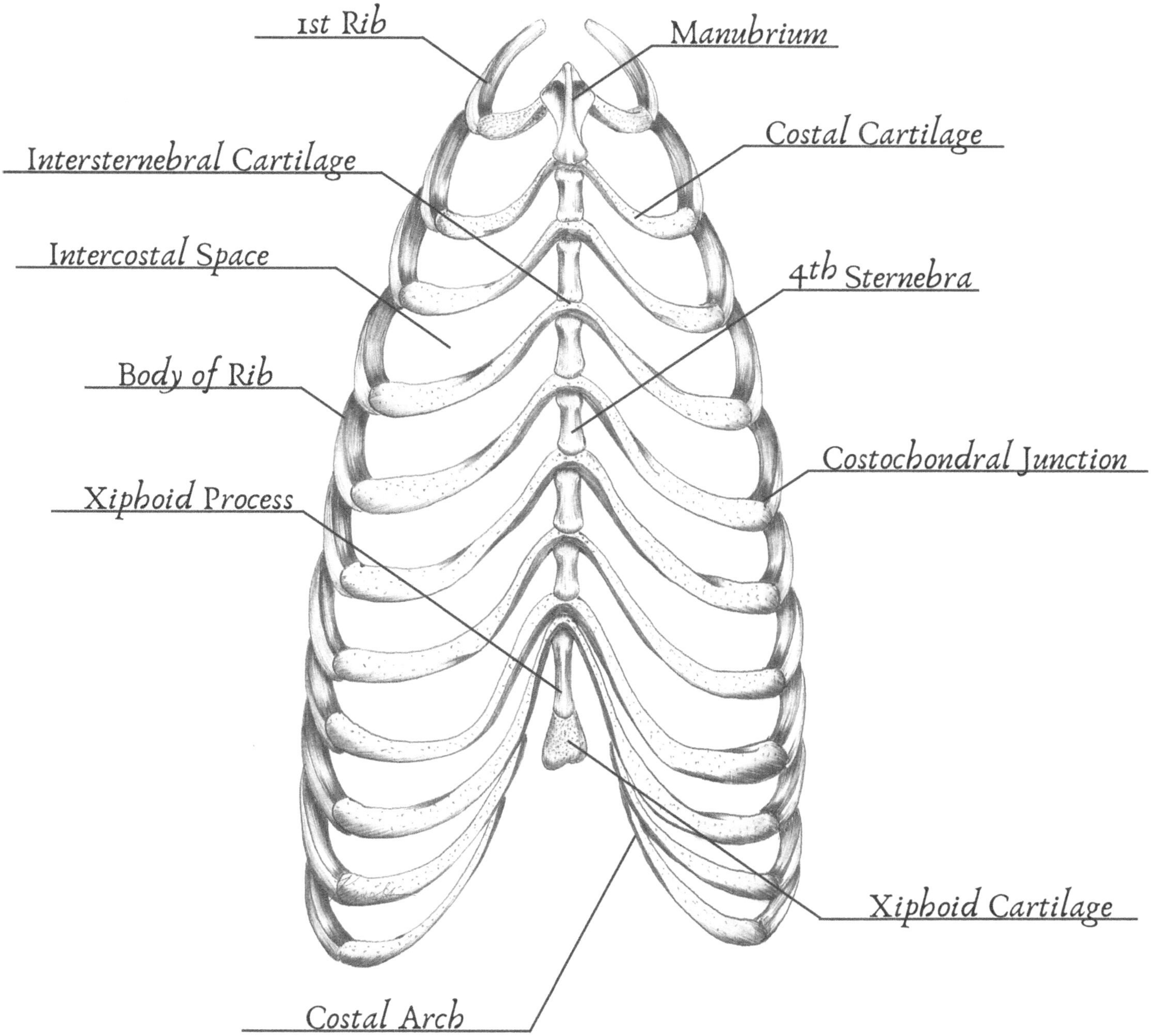

*T12 & T13 *floating ribs not included**

Ribs & Sternum: Anterior View

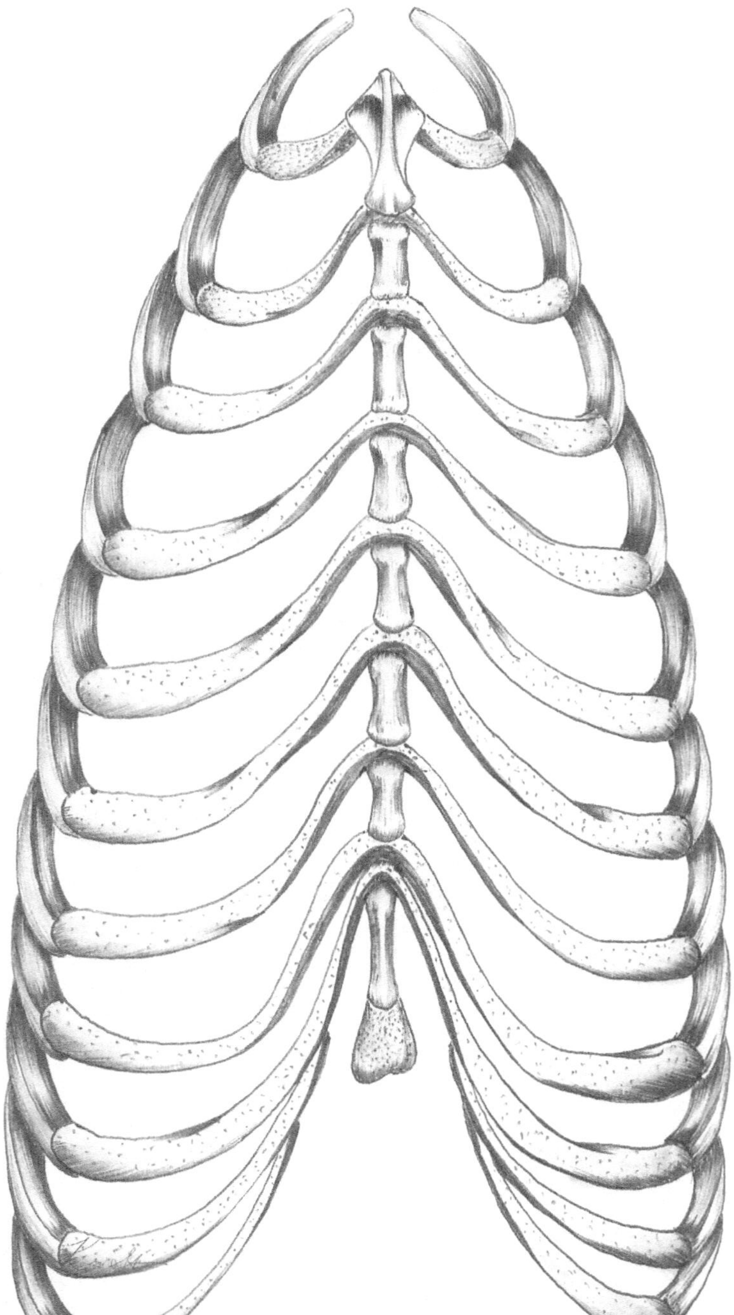

Respiratory System / Lungs

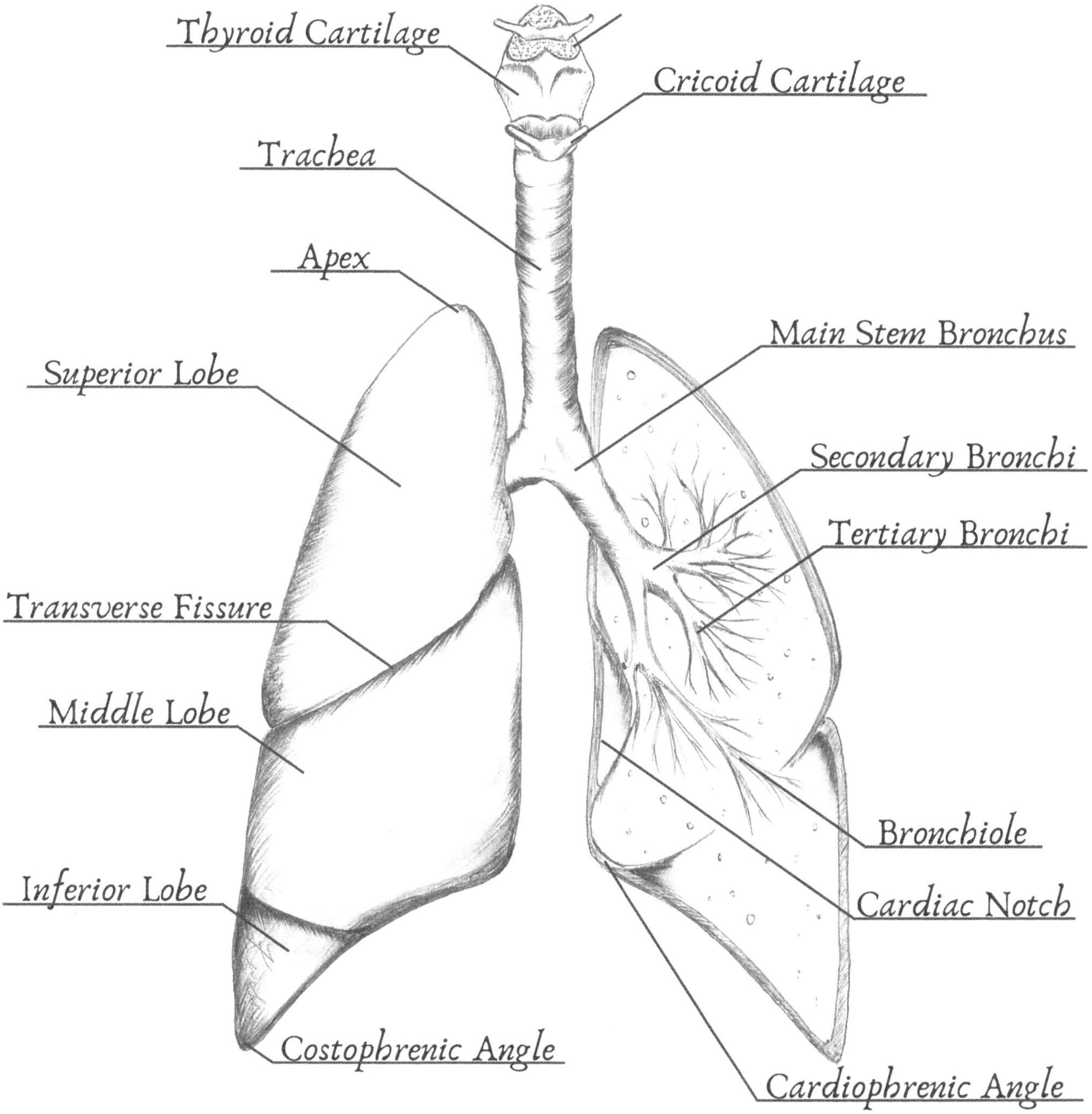

Respiratory System / Lungs

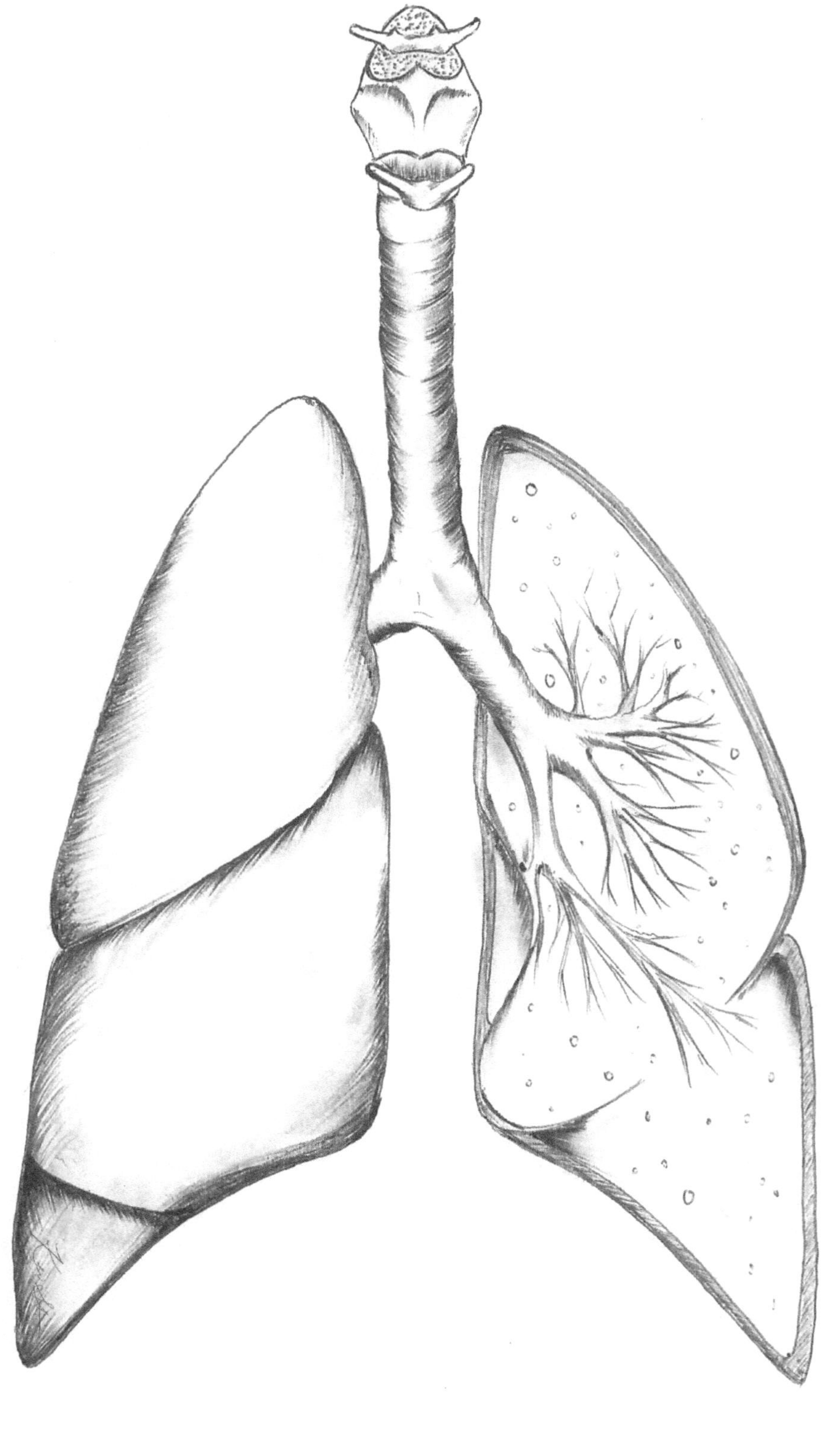

Heart: Anterior View

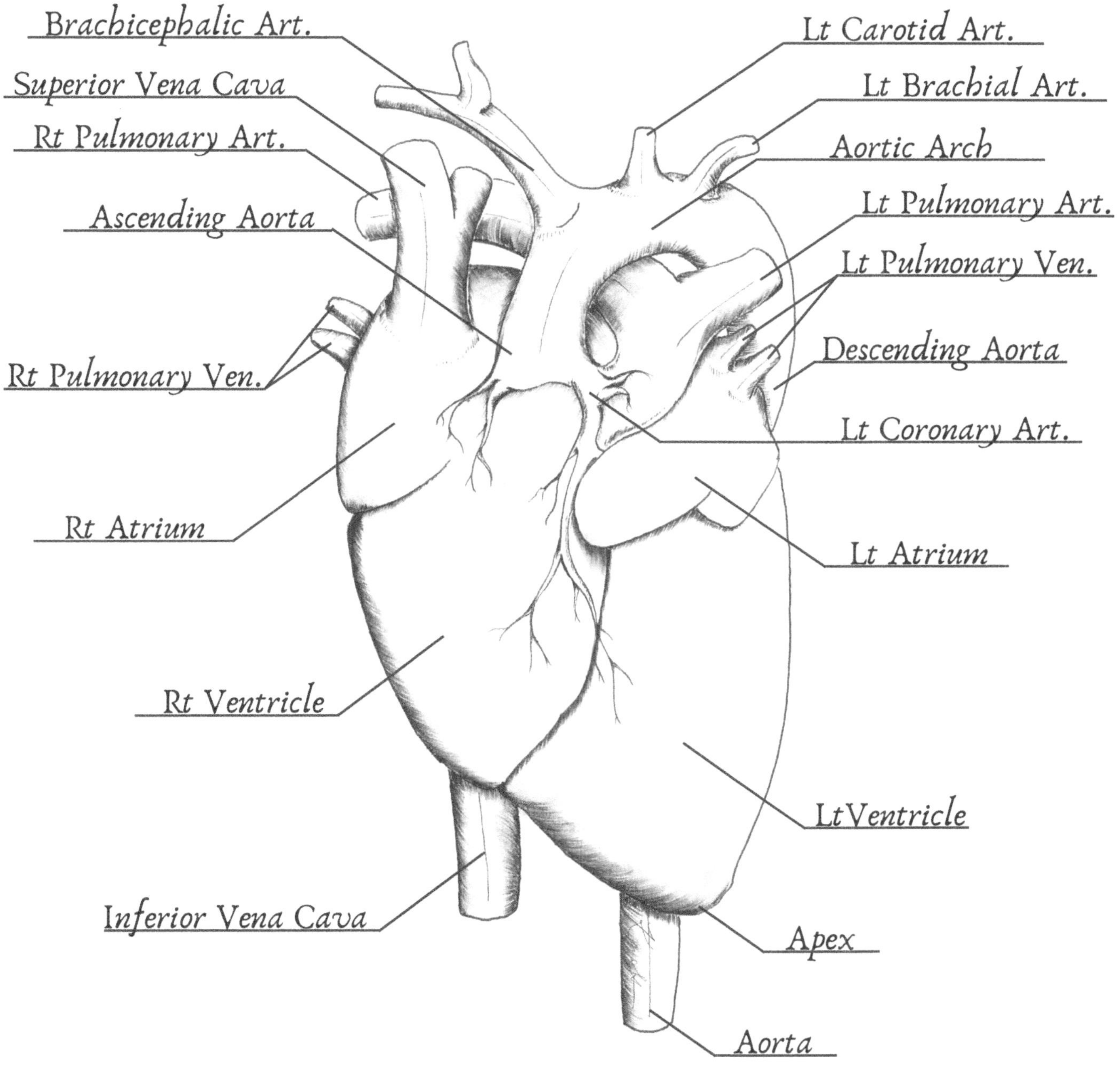

Heart: Anterior View

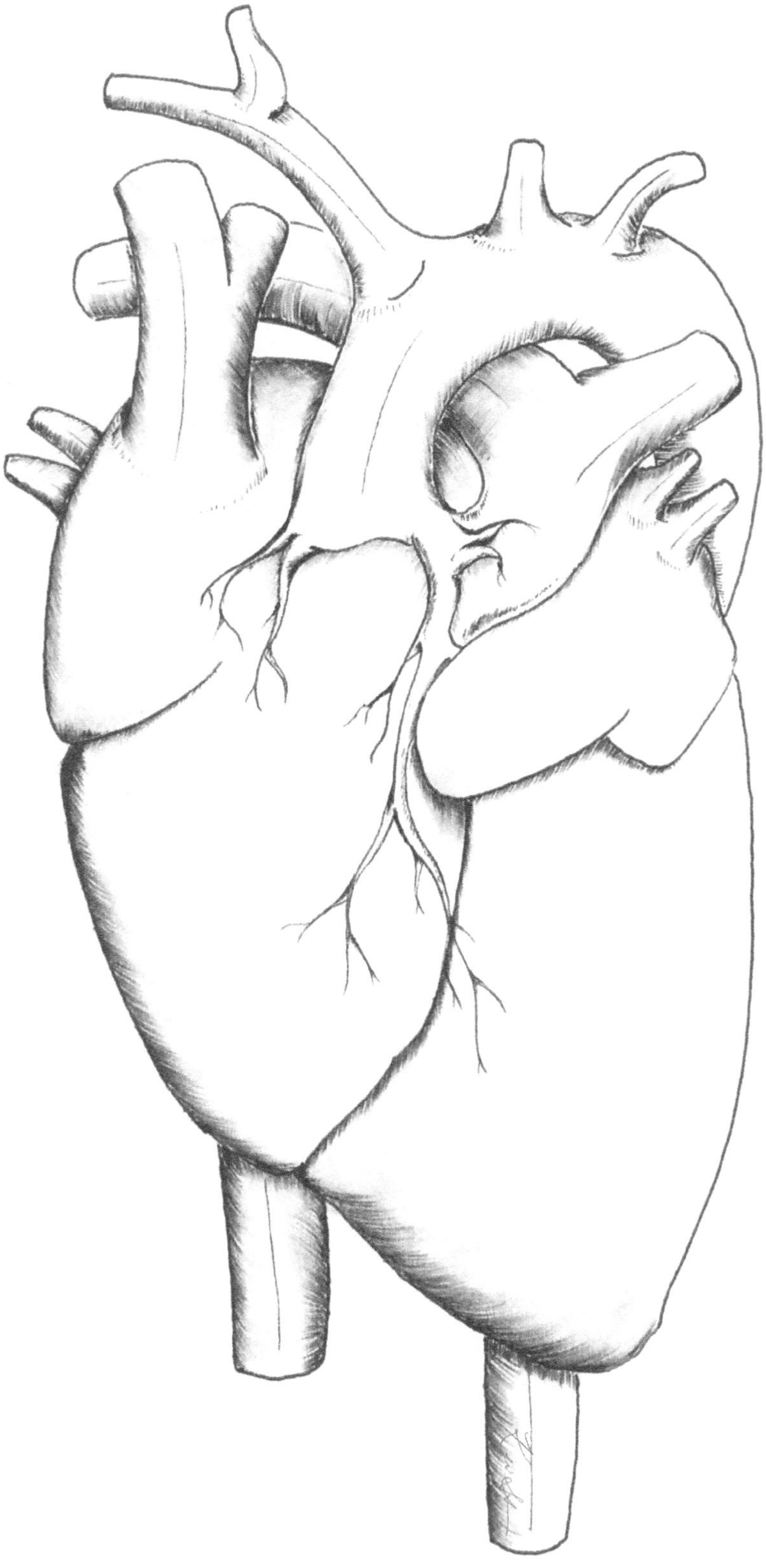

Heart: Dissected View

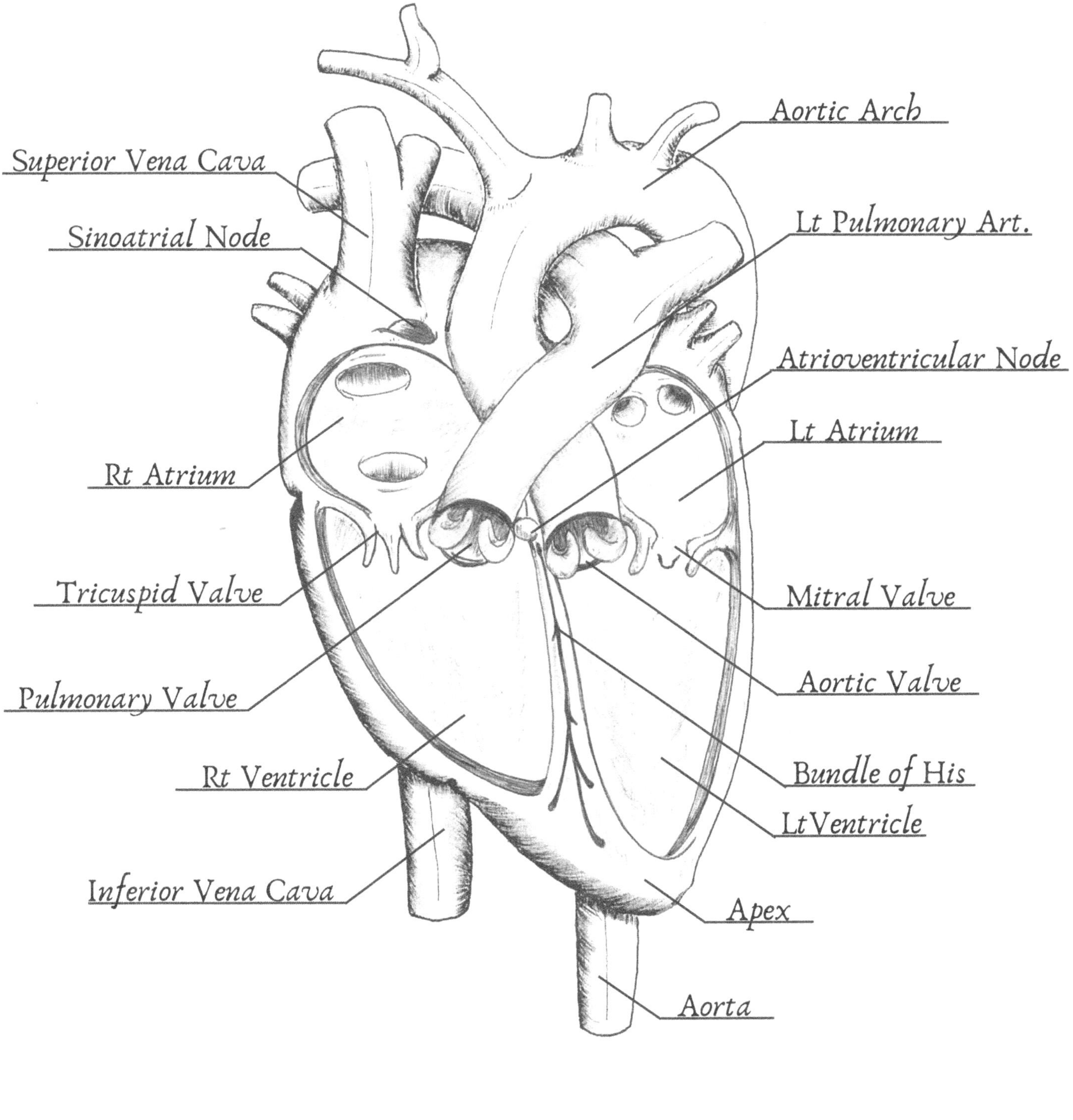

Heart: Dissected View

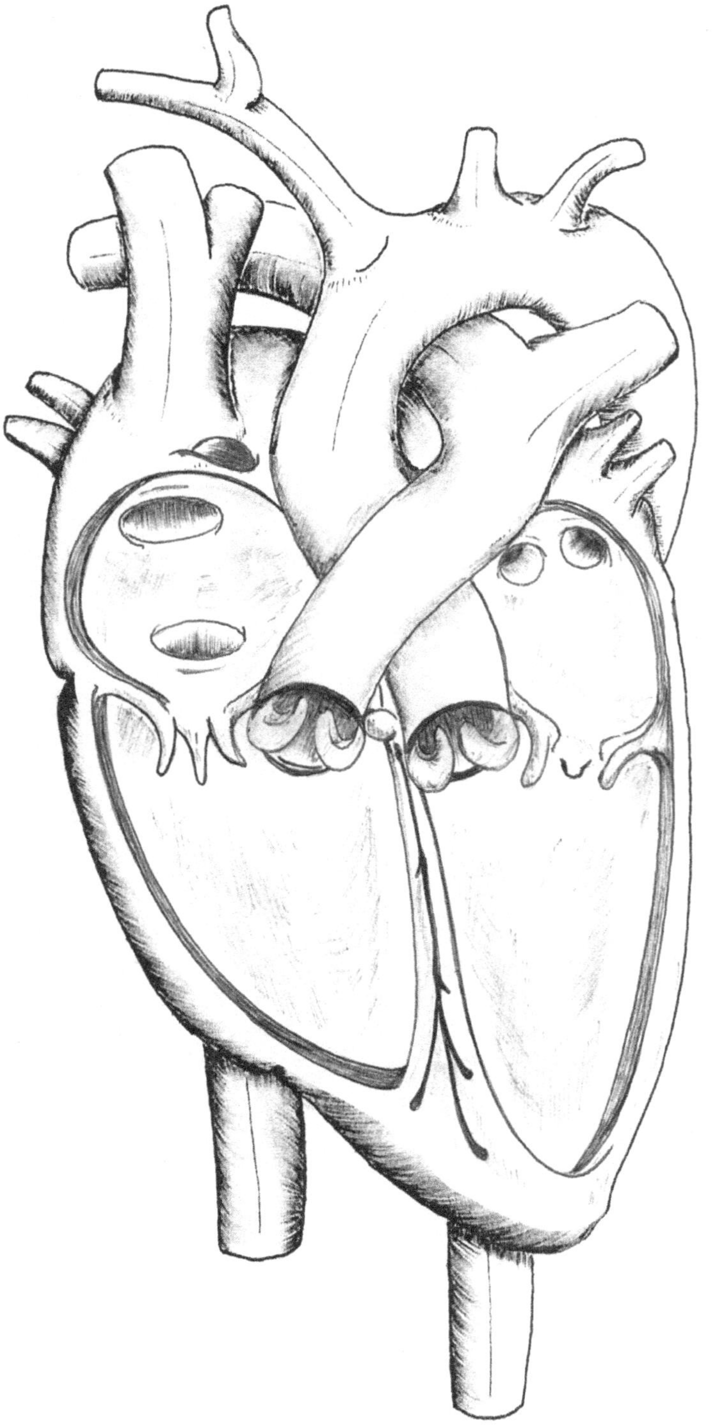

the Abdomen

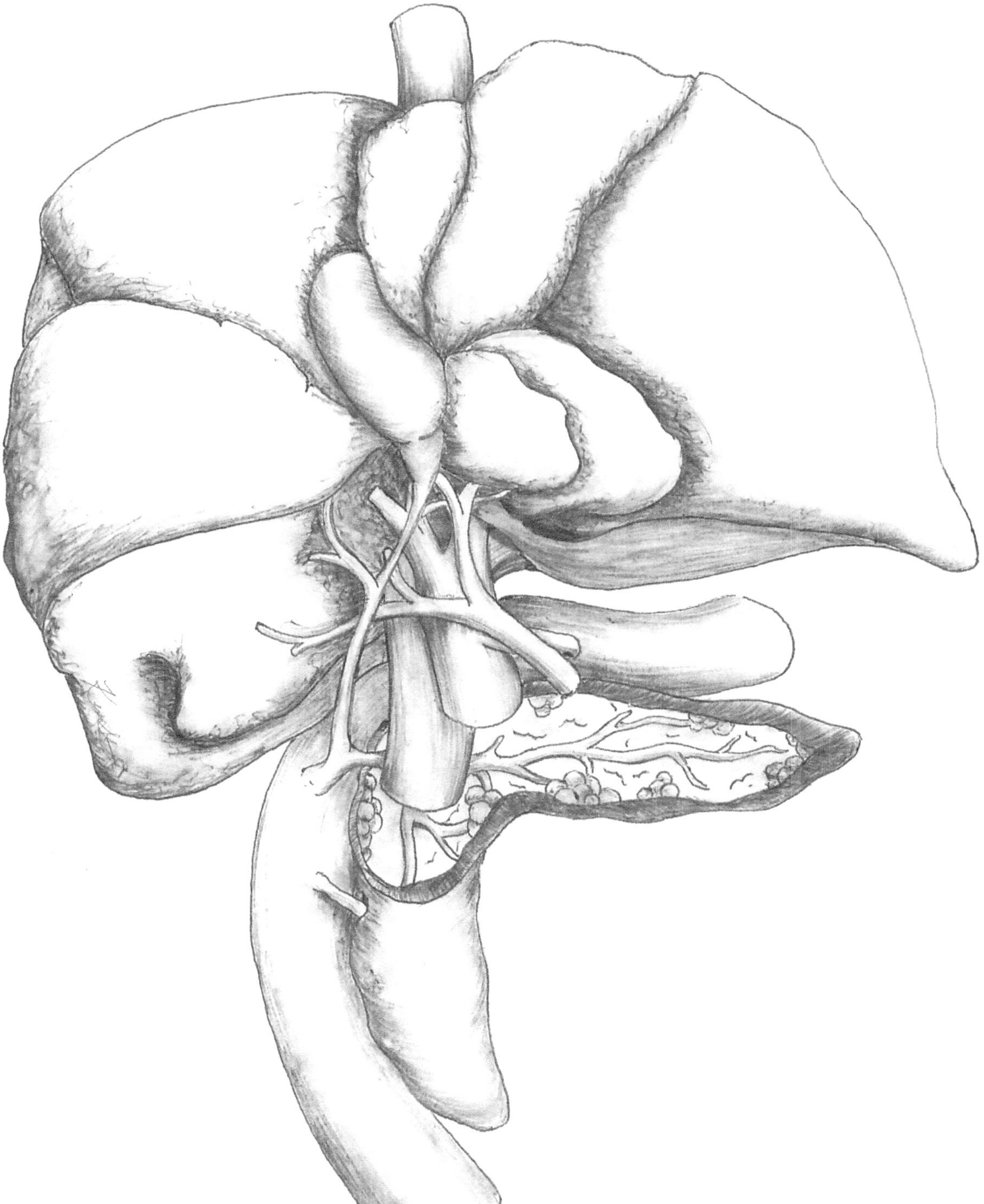

Notes:

- The abdominal cavity contains 7 major organs: the liver, spleen, pancreas, gall bladder, kidneys, and bladder. (not including the reproductive organs)
- The digestive system is comprised of the esophagus, stomach, small intestine, large intestine, rectum, and anus.
- The digestive system is roughly 3 times the length of the body.
- The gastric rugae are folds of tissue in the mucosa of the stomach providing elasticity for expansion and contraction of the stomach.
- The right kidney is positioned more cranially in the abdominal cavity than the left kidney.
- The liver is comprised of 6 lobes. left lateral (LL), left medial (LM), quadrate (Q), right medial (RM), right lateral (RL), caudate (C)
- The pancreas is a bi-lobed organ which contains groups of cells called the Islets of Langerhans which secrete insulin and glucagon.

Abdominal Arteries: Anterior View

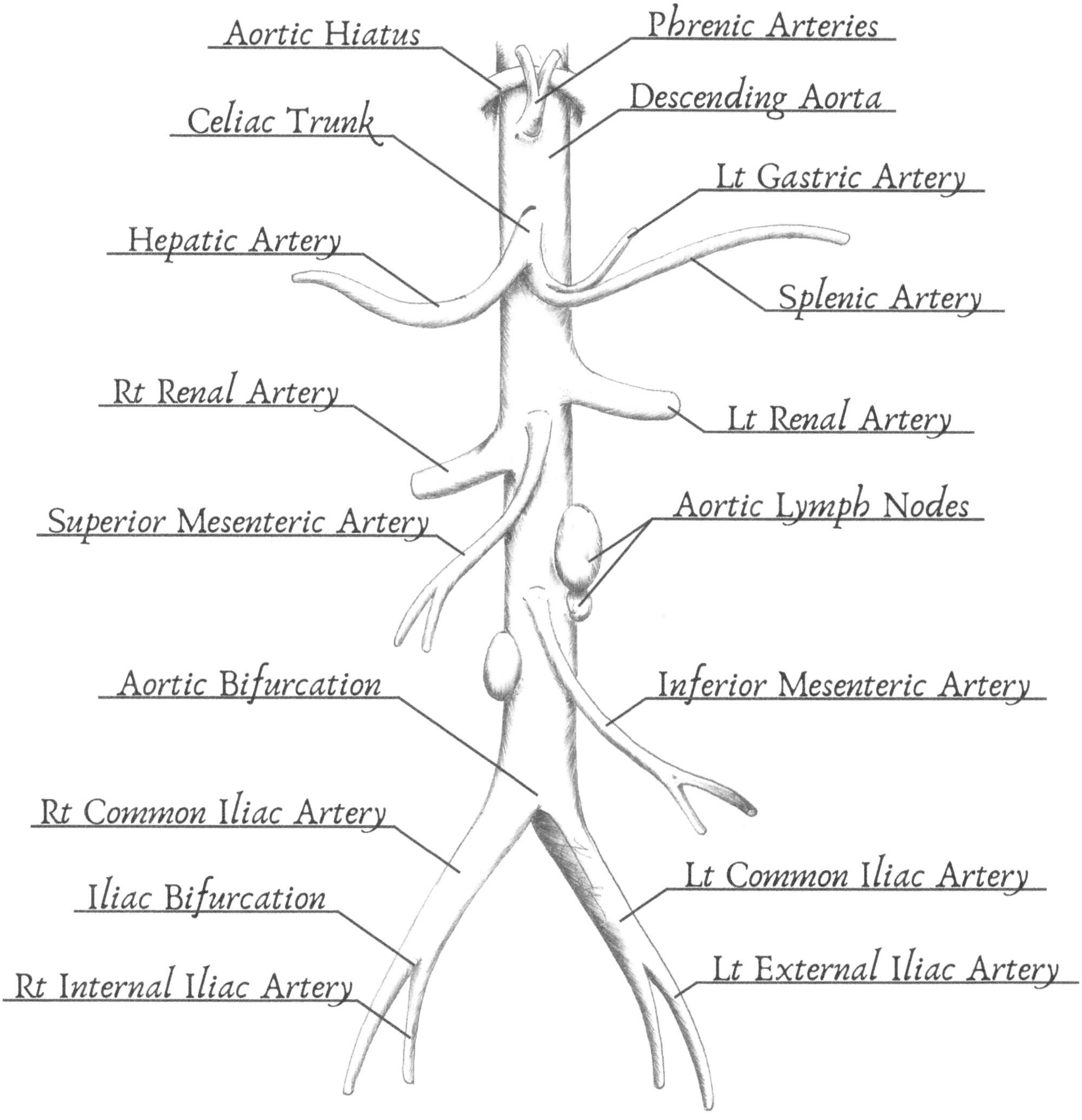

Abdominal Arteries: Anterior View

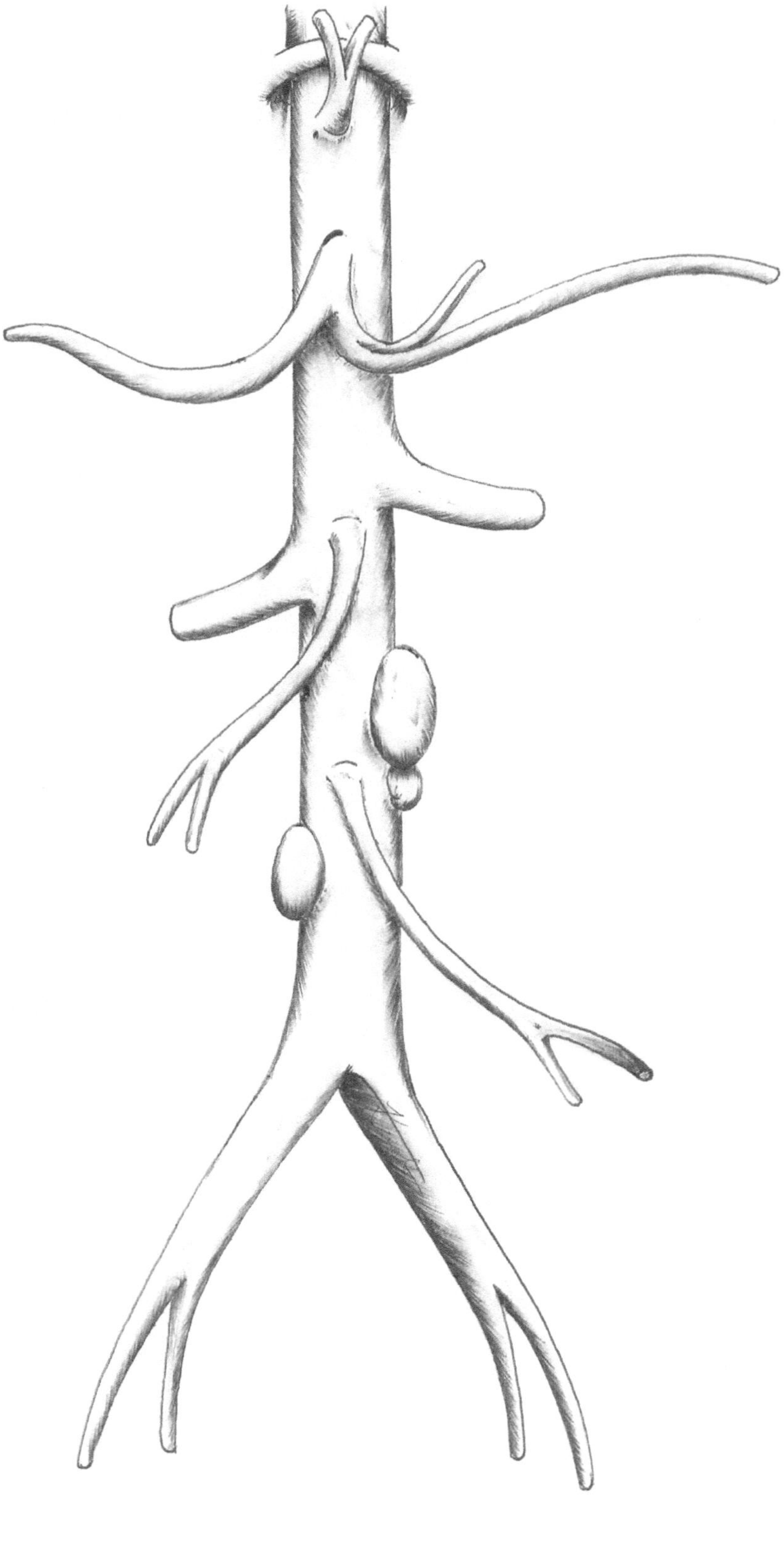

Liver & Biliary System

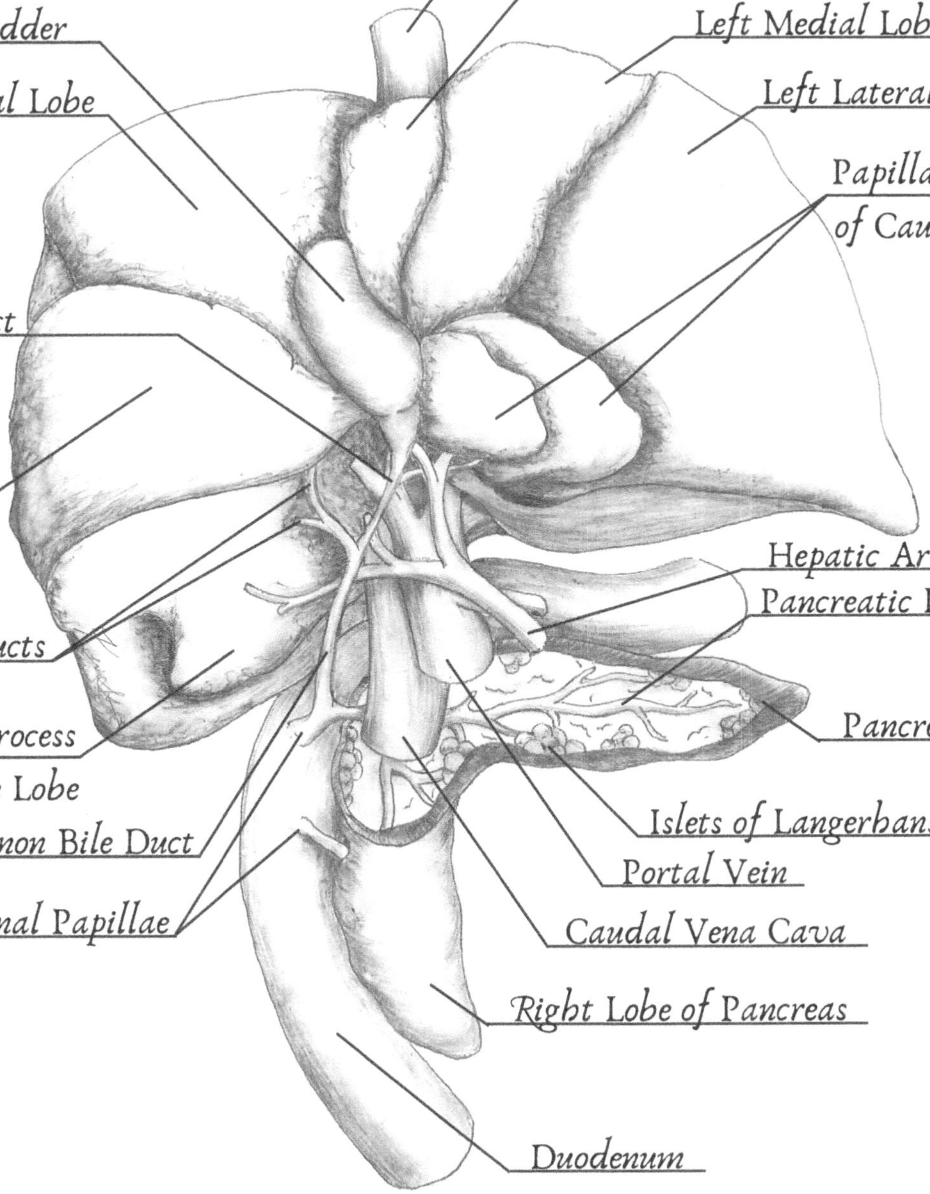

Liver & Biliary System

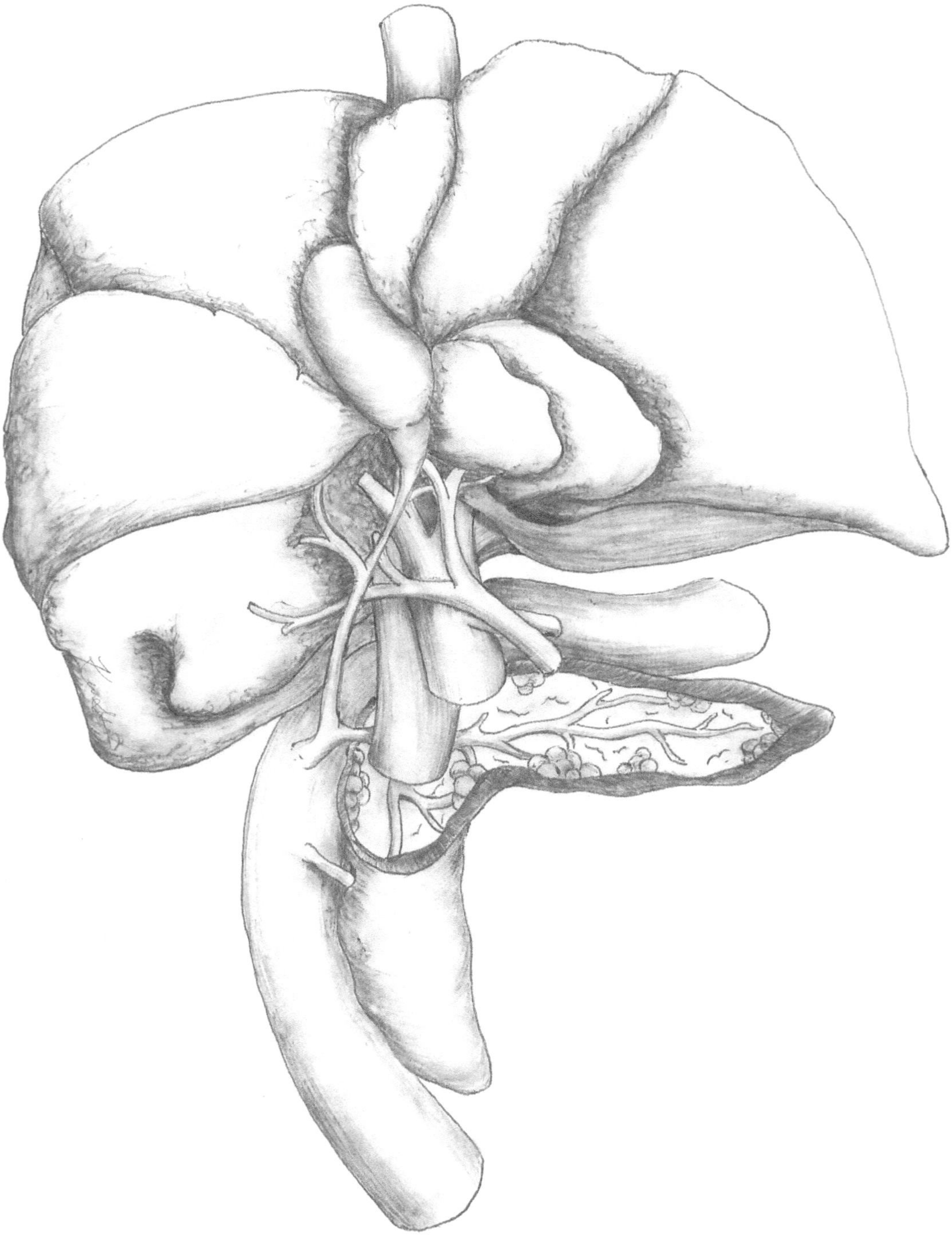

Gastrointestinal Tract: Anterior View

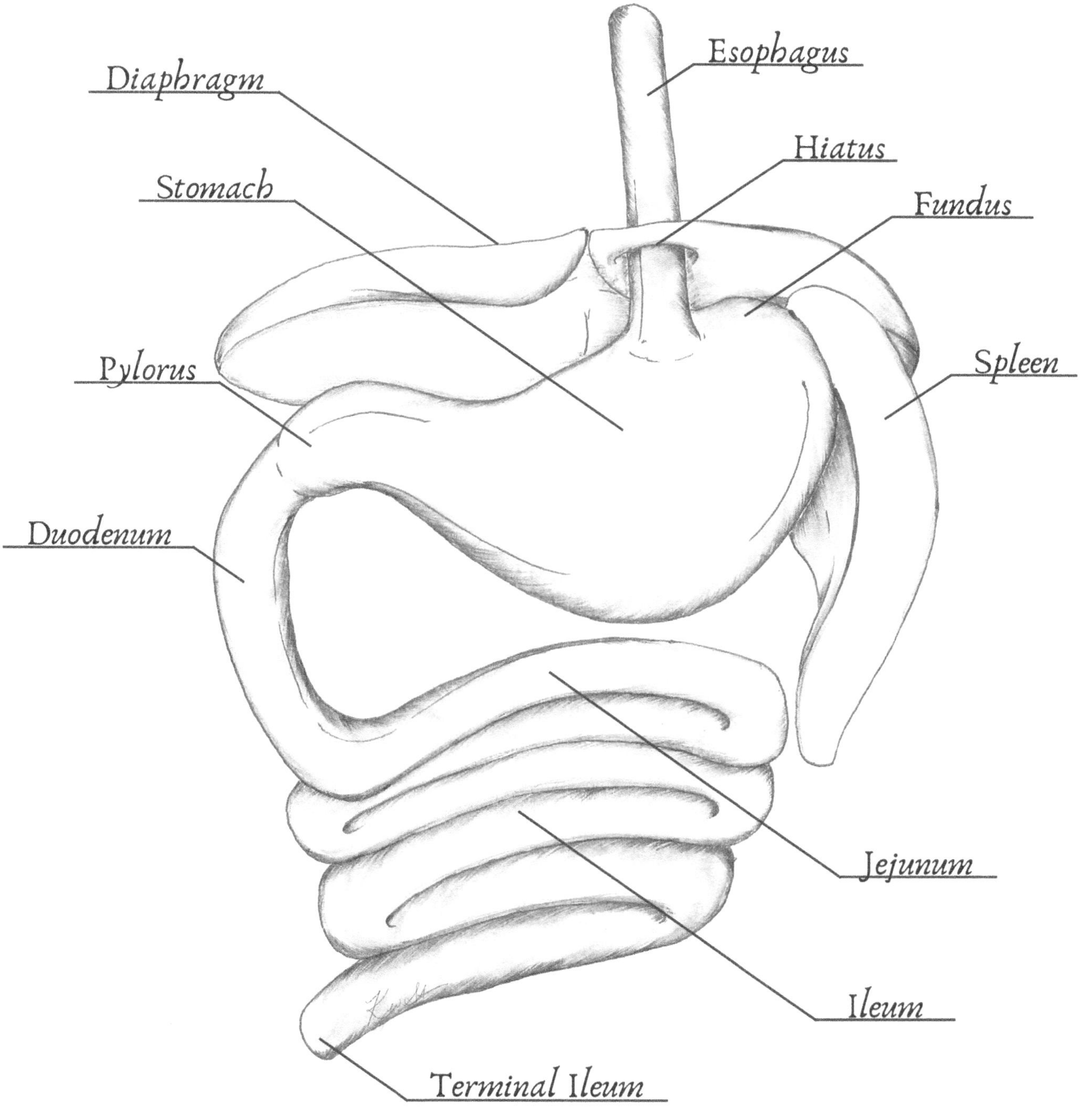

Gastrointestinal Tract: Anterior View

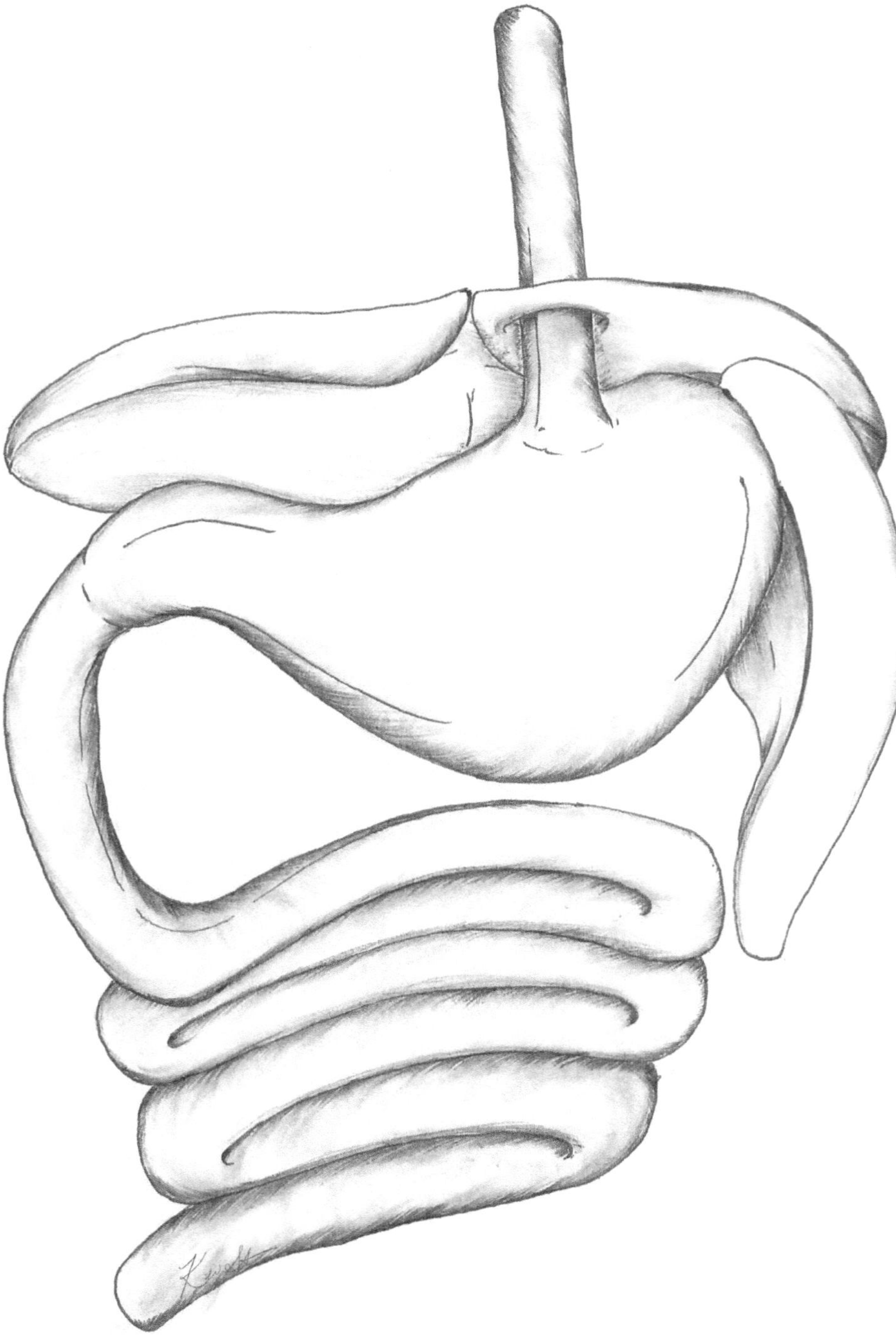

Large Intestine: Anterior View

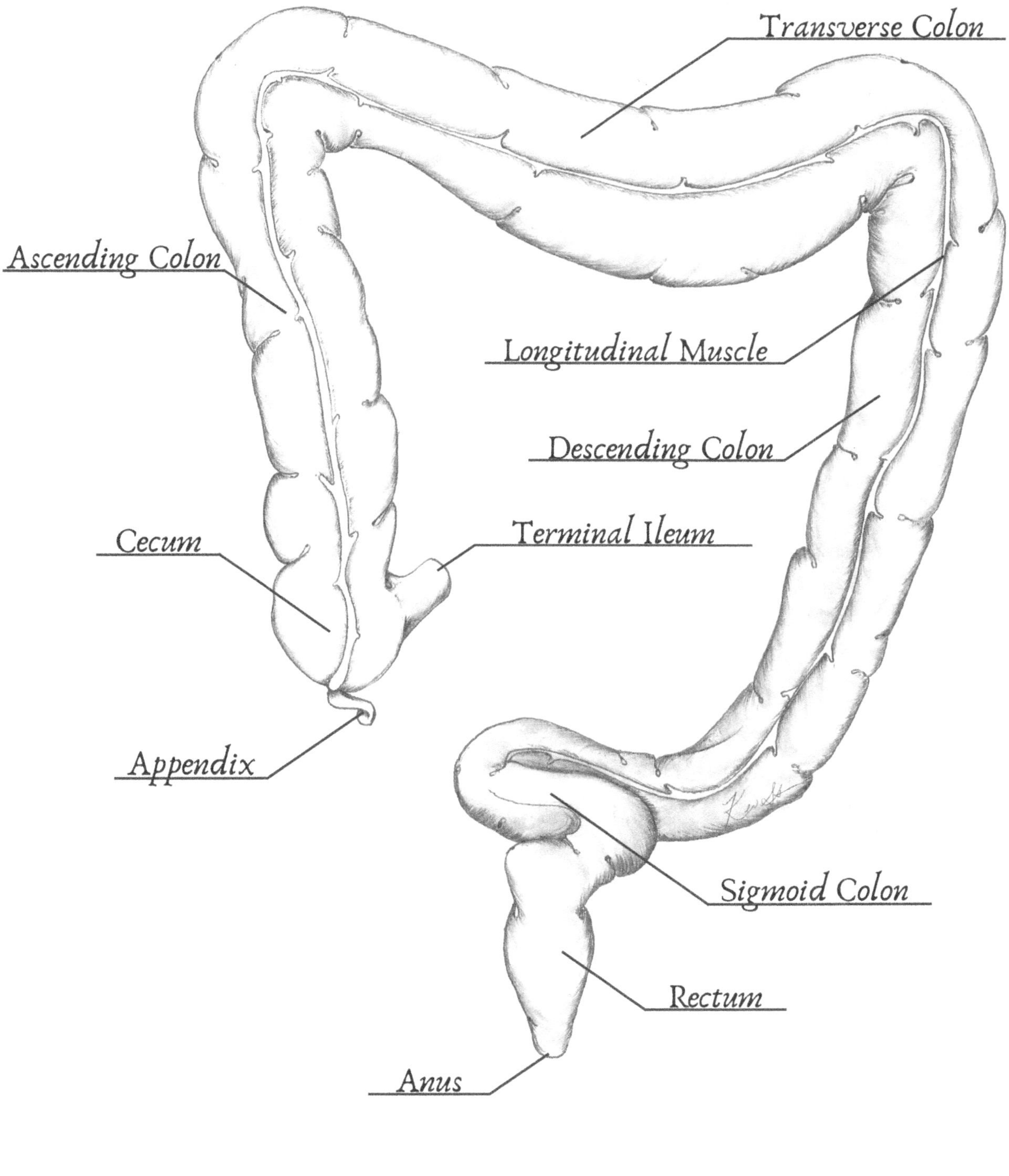

Large Intestine: Anterior View

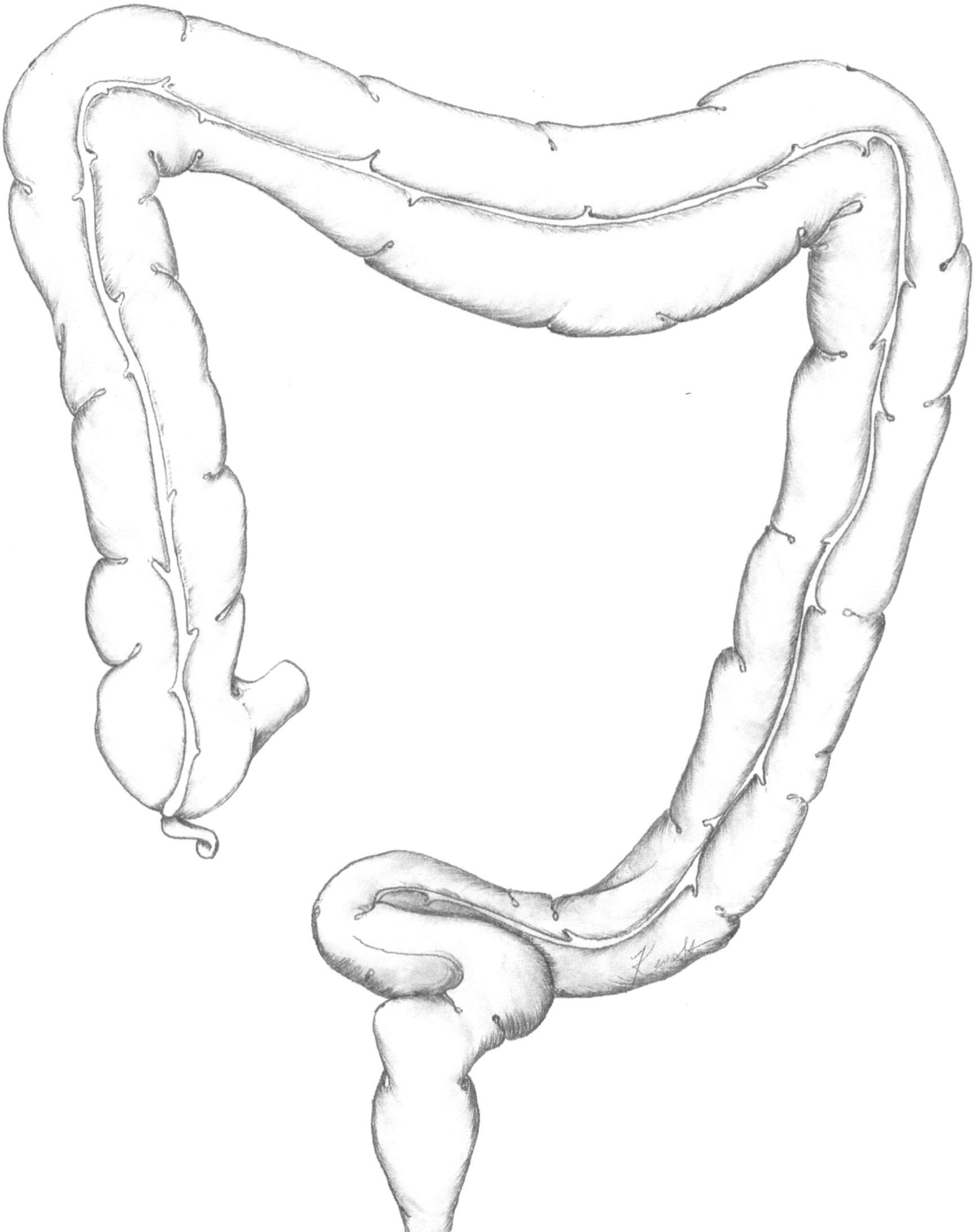

Kidney: Dissected View

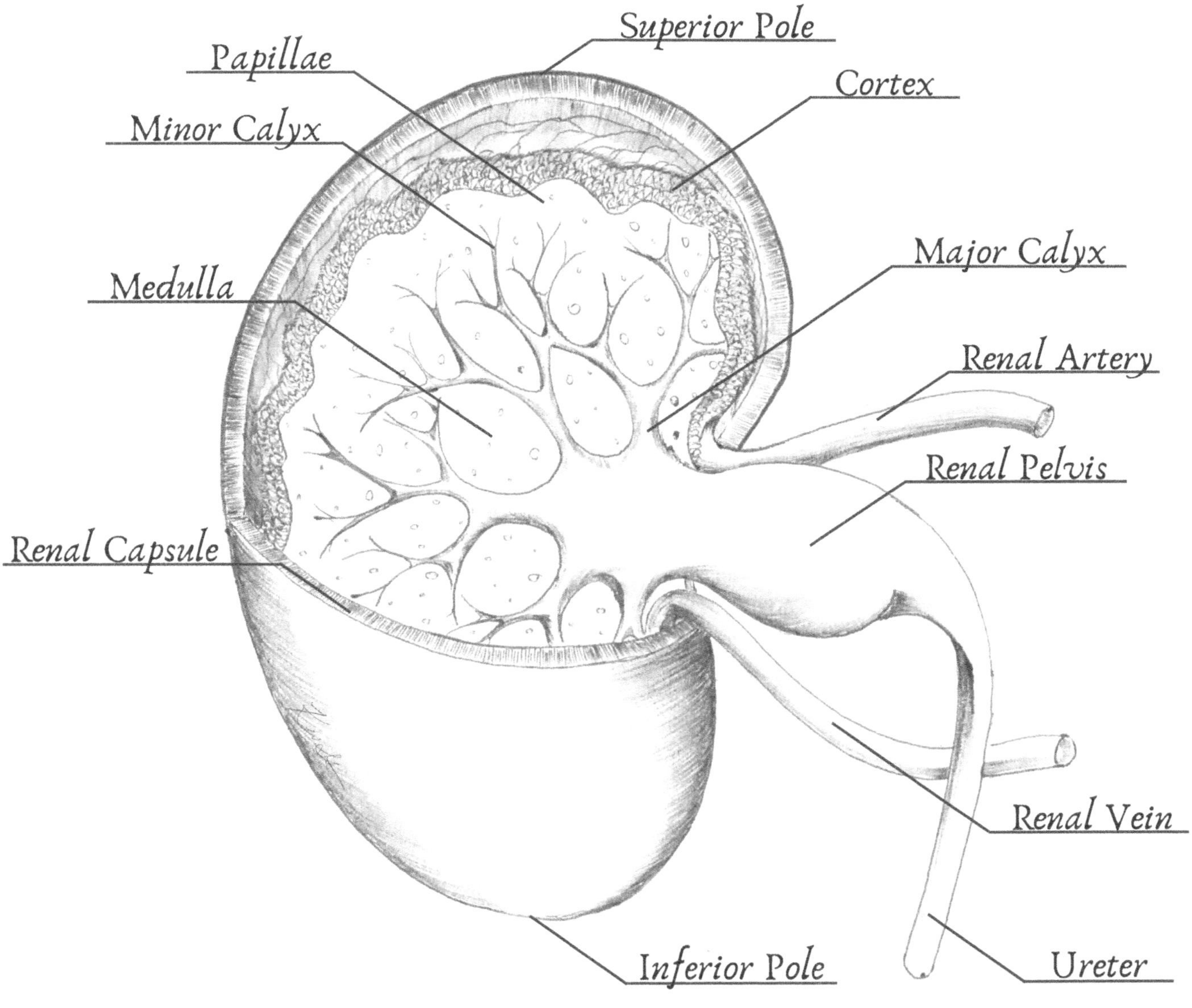

Kidney: Dissected View

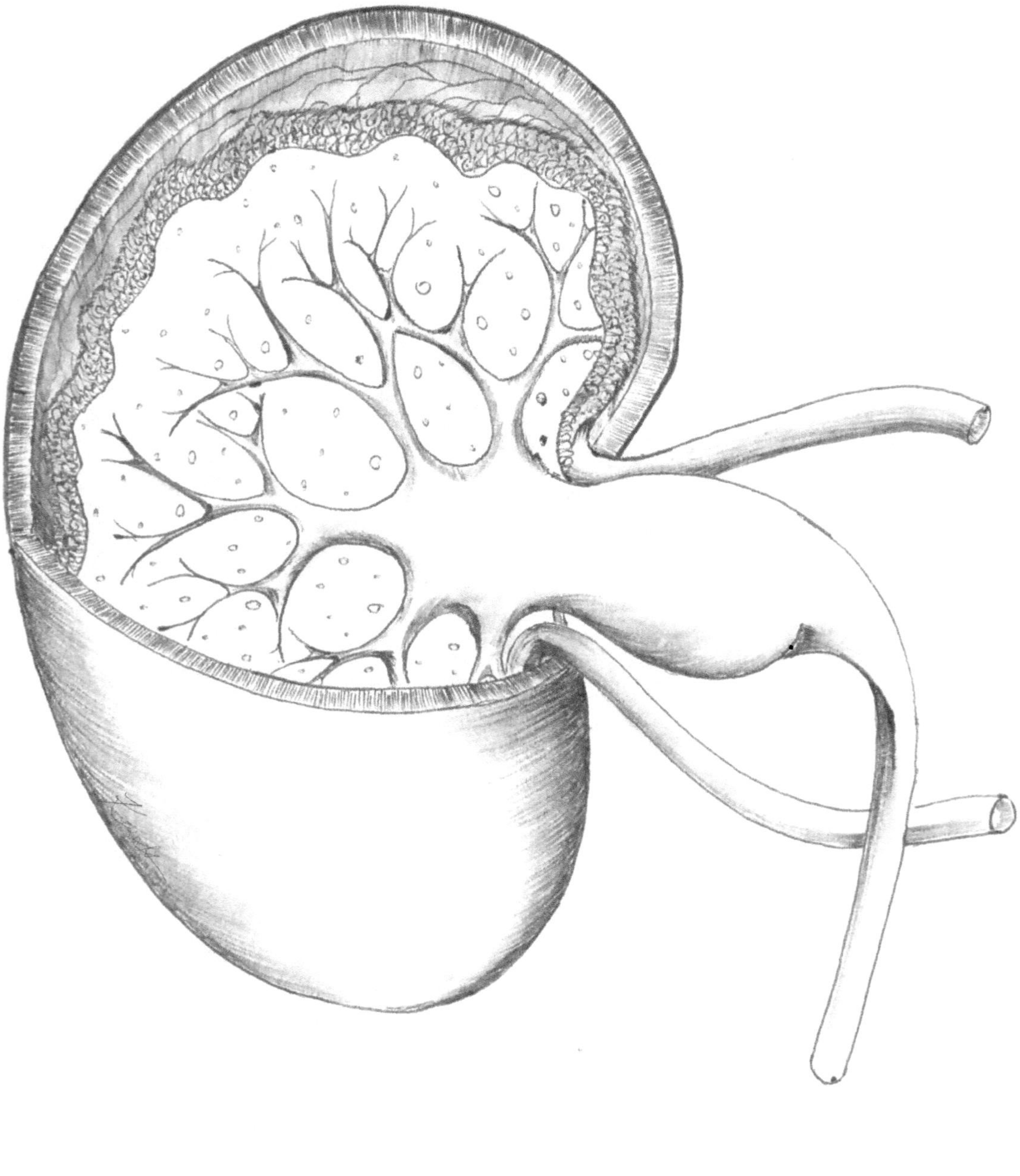

Urinary System

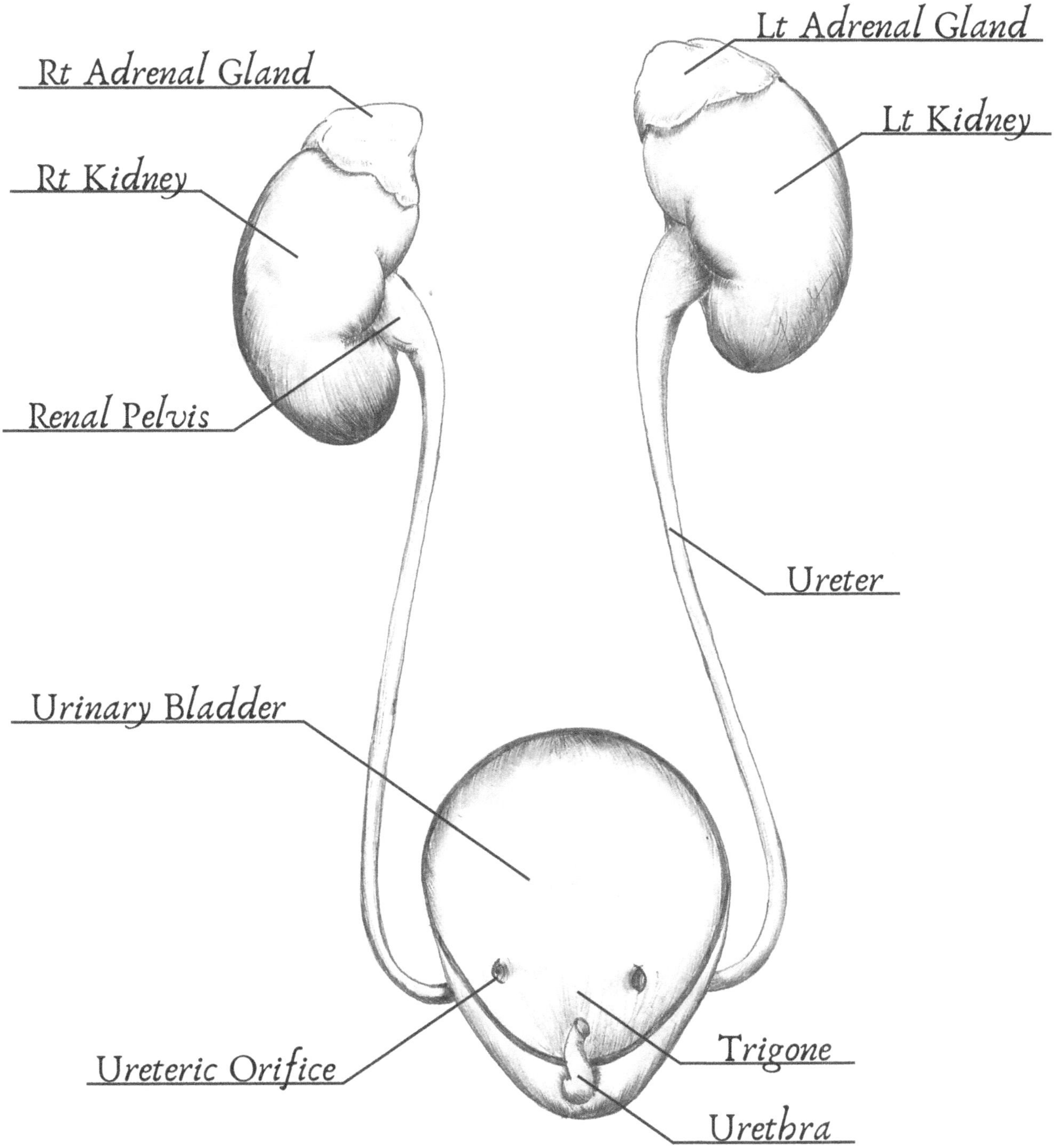

Urinary System

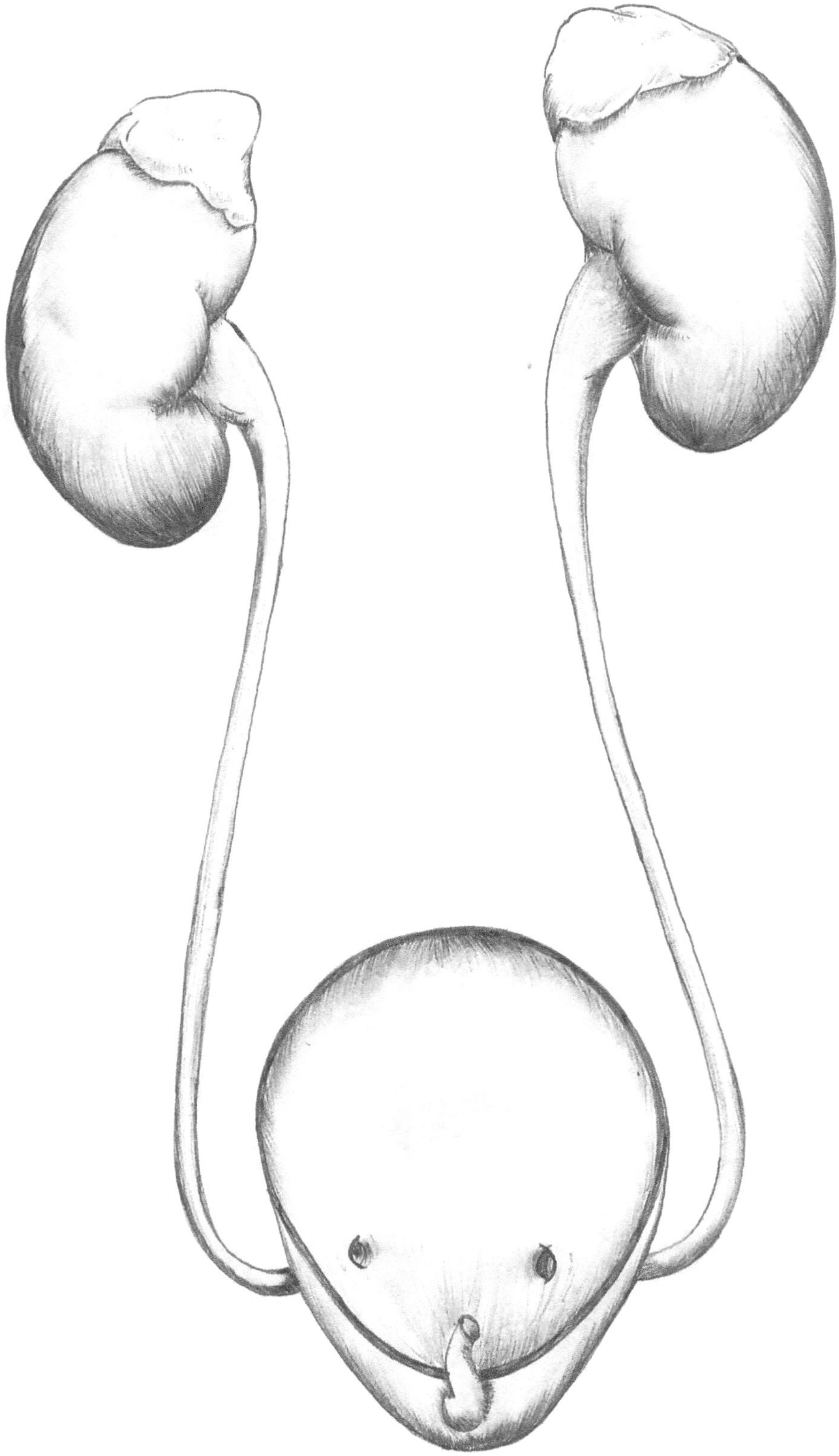

Reproductive System: Male

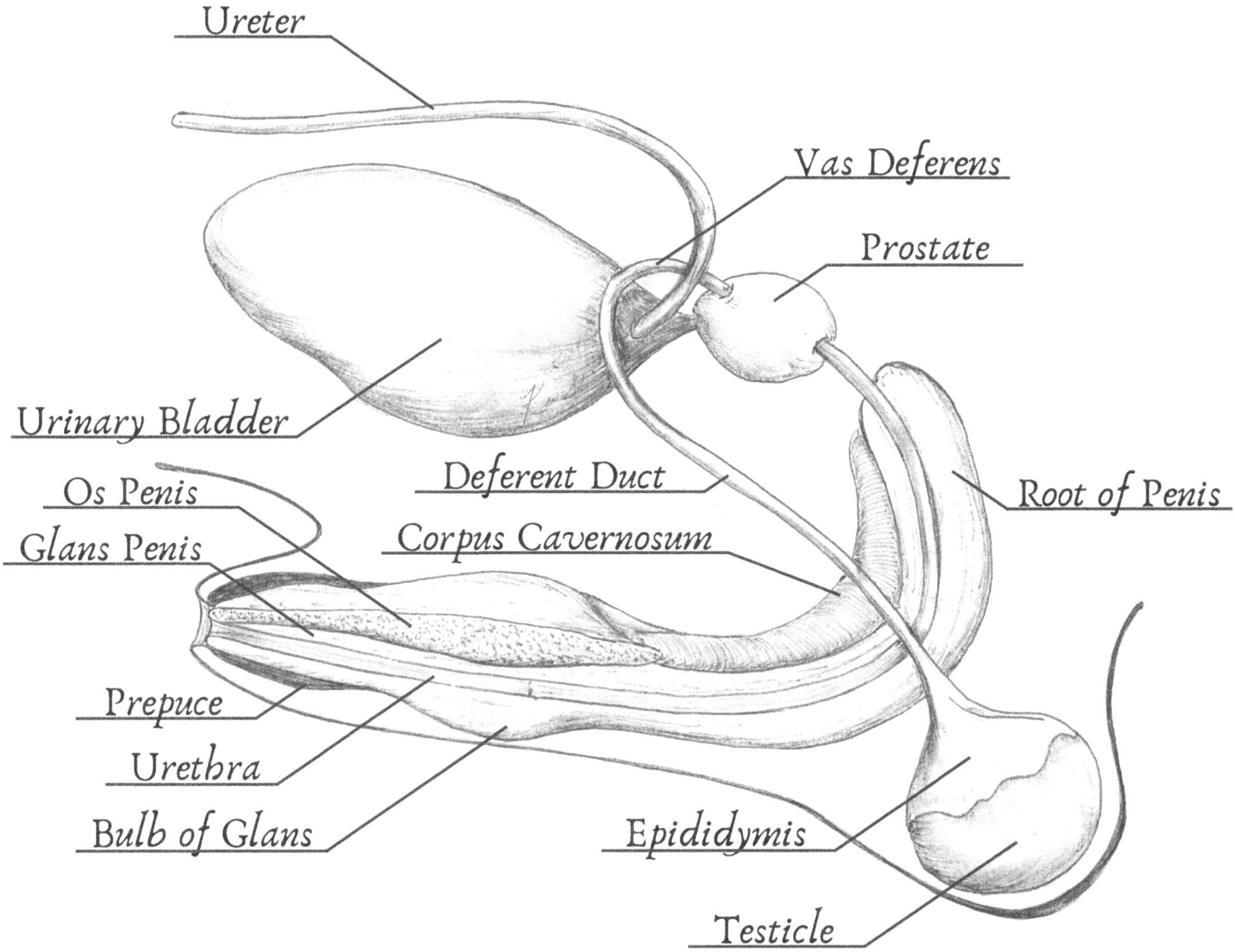

Reproductive System: Male

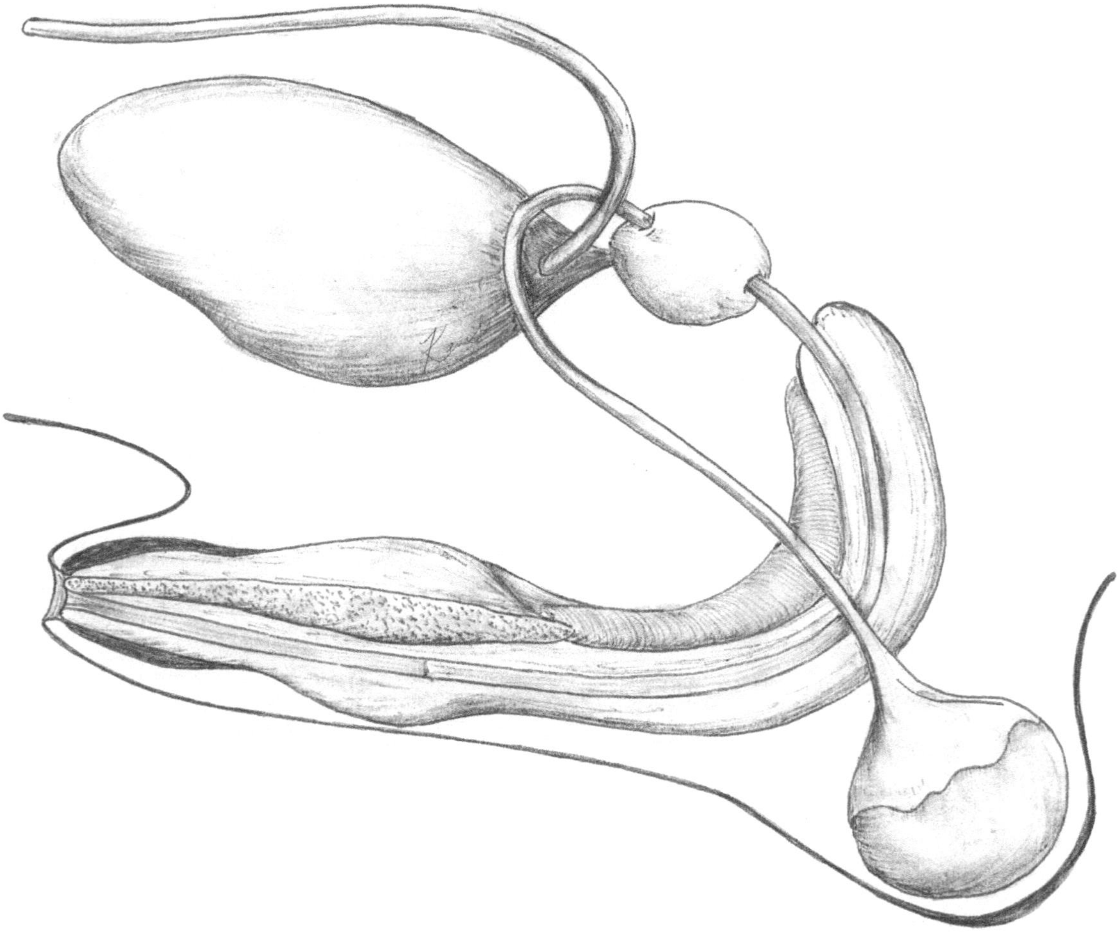

Reproductive System: Female

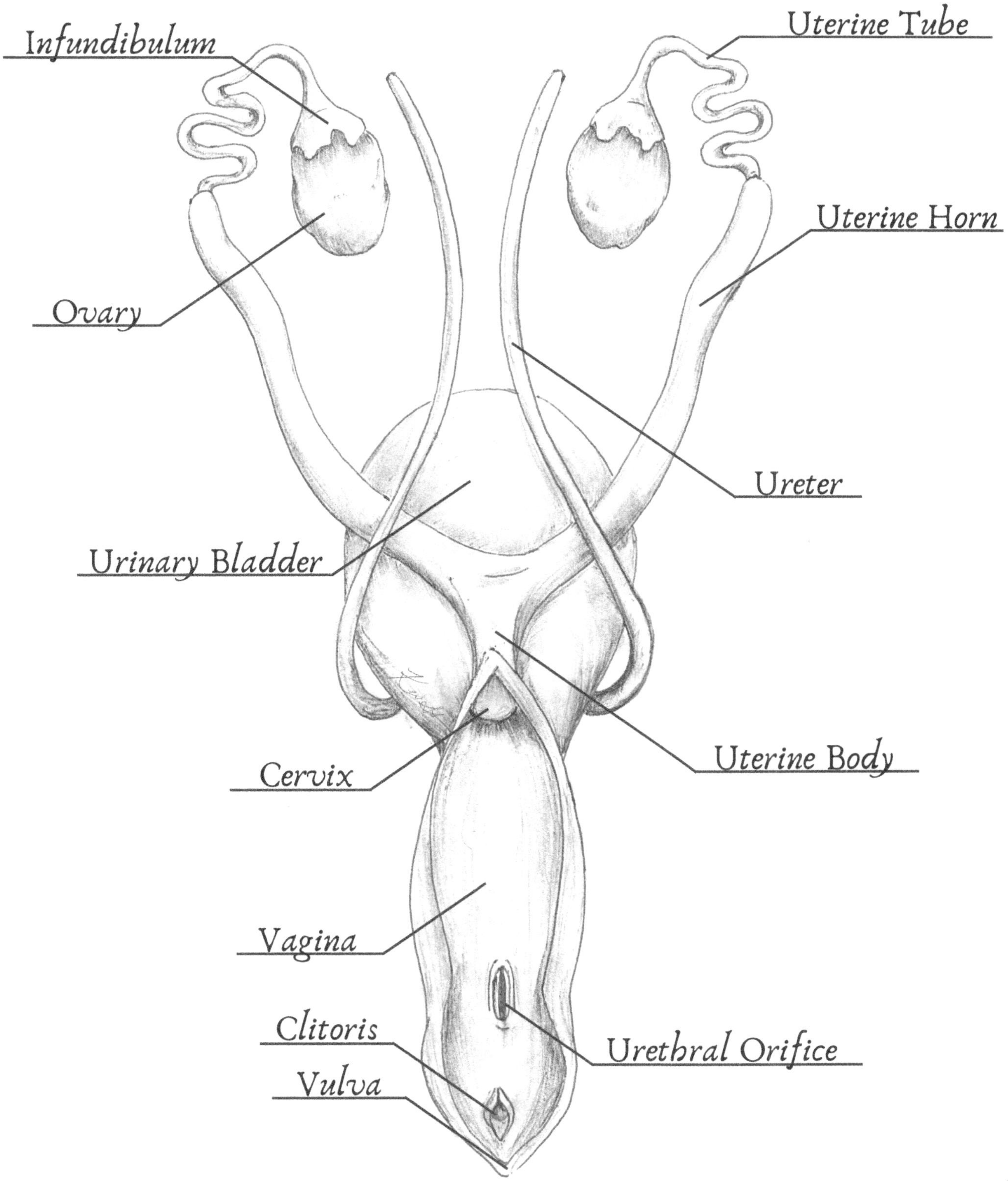

Reproductive System: Female

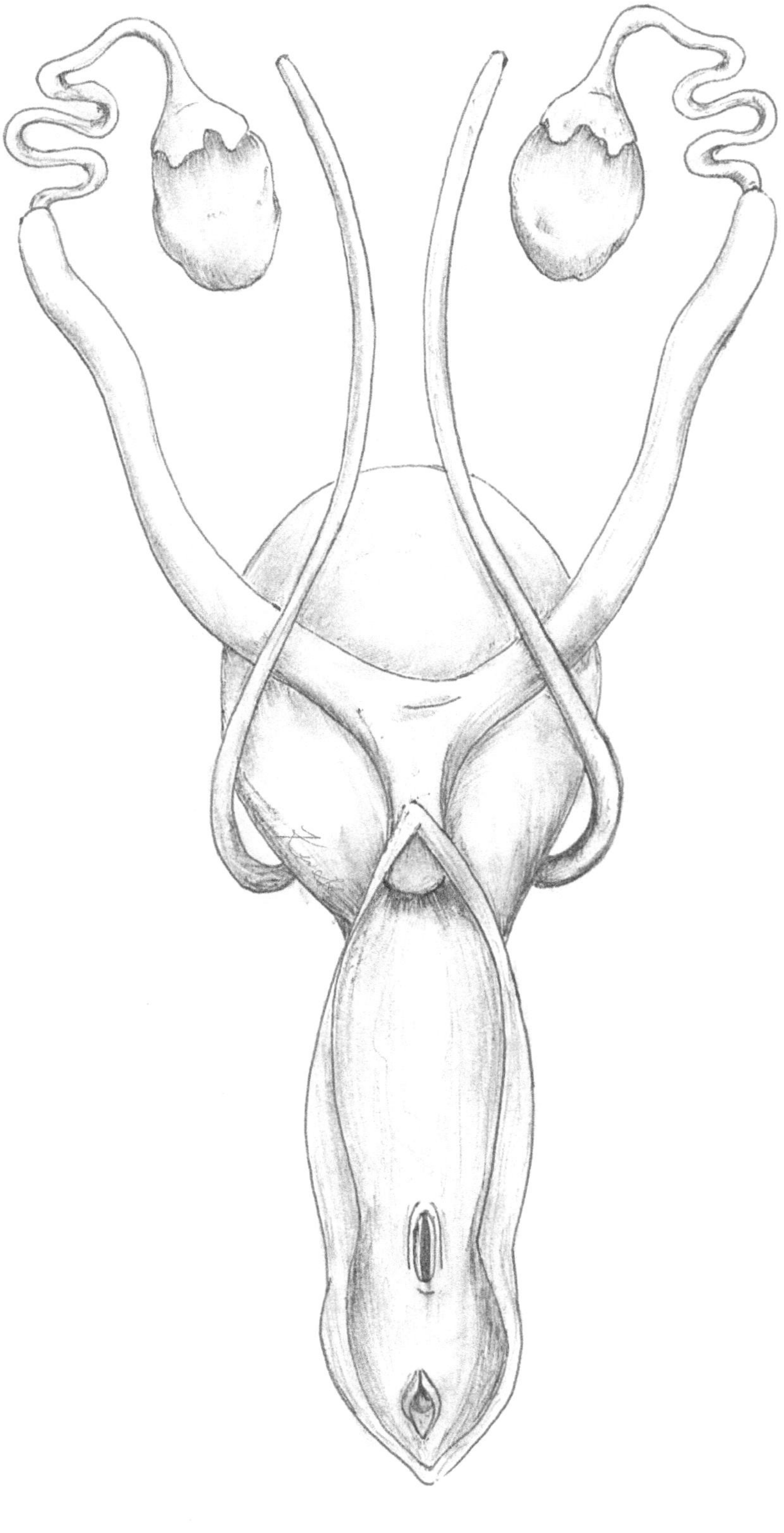

Index:

Index:

Index:

About the Author

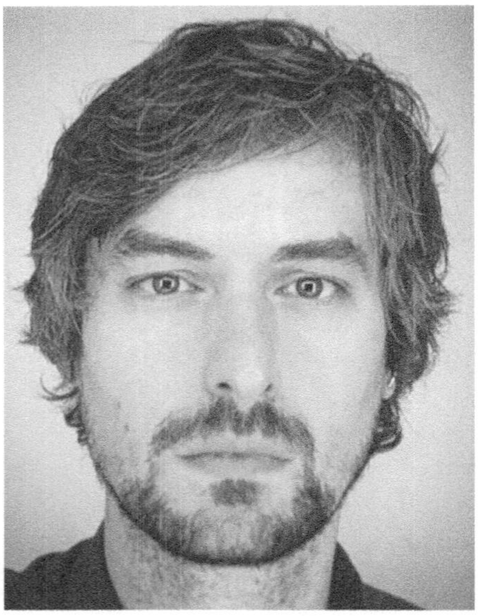

Kevin Stevens is a registered Radiographer and Magnetic Resonance Imaging Technologist. He has worked in medical imaging since 2002 and started work in veterinary medicine in 2009. Kevin is also a musician and an artist with a love for teaching. He is always looking for creative outlets in his career and in opportunities to share his knowledge with those around him. Originally from the United States, Kevin now resides with his wife and children in Ottawa, Ontario, Canada.

Kevin is also the creator of V.I.R.A, the veterinary imaging resource academy, a free online resource for veterinary imaging personnel. For More information about veterinary imaging or to reach Kevin please visit **www.vet-image.com**

Made in United States
Cleveland, OH
05 November 2026

47664131R00063